Fake Diseases

By Ryan Aleckszander

Written in 2021
Kirkland Lake, Ontario
Canada

Cover art by Ryan Alecksžander

www.NotusBooks.org

Updated in March 2022

1. What is Disease?

I think the word "disease" is misleading. Even when taken literally, as a lack of ease, or a lack of health, it doesn't seem to help us much to think about health problems in terms of "disease."

(noun) Disease

> early 14c., "discomfort, inconvenience, distress, trouble", from Old French desaise "lack, want; discomfort, distress; trouble, misfortune; disease, sickness", from des- "without, away"

The root of the word doesn't seem to help us. Likely, if you are experiencing a health problem, you already understand that it is troubling. It doesn't really help to have a doctor give you a Latin name for it, especially if the only treatments involved are some kind of pharmaceutical drug, surgery, or test.

As "alternative" practitioners, we are in a tricky situation. In most cases, we're not legally allowed to "treat" any diseases. Strictly, in most cases we're not legally allowed to "treat" people.

We are allowed to "support and promote the maintenance and repair of a healthy body." It's not as jazzy as talking about diseases and "cures", but most curiously in this language, we learn that medical doctors (MDs) themselves hardly talk of "cures" at all either.

There are runs and walks for the cures. There are all types of fundraisers that use the word of a disease next to the word "cure". But you probably won't find many medical professionals willing to use the word.

Once I boarded a tightly packed caravan from California to Mexico. We were on our way to a seminar that I was to co-host. I shook the hand of the man next to me, and I asked what he does. He responded enthusiastically: "I cure people of chronic diseases."

His response illustrates perfectly why so many people are willing to travel to "lesser" countries for "medical tourism." They can at least get real answers in plain English.

It seems most people really don't know that a medical doctor is not trained in curing diseases. They *are* trained in "treating" diseases. "Managing" is the current word. Many are also trained in a specialty, such as surgery, anesthesiology, pathology, etc. But it is all under the "disease management" umbrella, with the exception of infectious diseases, which I will cover as well.

The language defines the practice. As alternative practitioners, it is lucky for us that we are not allowed to "treat diseases", because that's not really what we want to do. And we don't treat people for problems. We don't support problems, we "support and promote the maintenance and repair of a healthy body." A healthy body does not have a "disease." A healthy body does not have a discomfort, a trouble (physical, at least), or a physical inconvenience. Still not very jazzy.

A lot of our work in dealing with people out in the wild, is rewiring how they think about disease. Daily, we are asked direct questions in the form of: "Can I cure this disease?"

Legally, I cannot answer this properly. But in this book I have attempted to deal with each category of disease, in simple language we can all understand.

I called this book *Fake Diseases* because this tangling of words is more than just not-helpful, it has trapped us in a system of medical thought and medical practice that makes it much less likely you will reach "ease", or health.

In the worst cases, the medical response to a disease can harm or kill a patient. Much of this is brushed off as an order of business. But in the alternative world, by aiming to support and promote maintenance and repair, then we are giving the body the ability to *heal itself.*

That last point there, "heal thyself," is truly an obscure term these days. In this post-2020 writing, surely all future readers know of the recent hysteria. Surely the words "heal thyself" were nowhere in the worldwide discussion. Somehow the human immune system, the system that deals with infectious threats, was almost entirely left out of the conversation. I am sure the average person knows that their body can overcome regular infections, but media hysteria failed to remind them.

This actually leads us to the premise, and the difference, between schools of medicine. Any medical field or "school" will fall into one of two categories: holistic, or allopathic. Holistic is sometimes spelled wholistic – implying the perspective of the whole body – and allopathic is sometimes called western medicine, conventional medicine, or orthodox medicine. That is a definition from Healthline.com. They say it can also be called biomedicine, or even mainstream medicine. The words really are informative, but if you didn't know the difference between holistic and allopathic, you'd think there is only one option for "treatment."

Allopathic MDs are really the only profession in the "mainstream" camp. Osteopaths are sometimes called allopathic, and sometimes they prefer to identify as holistic. The only real difference between the schools is the premise: the body can maintain and repair itself, or it is just waiting to break and in need of pharmaceutical or surgical intervention.

The allopathic school thinks that "disease" is a natural consequence of being alive, and that drugs or surgery are the best ways to "manage" this. The holistic schools, which is everyone else in the healing world, think that the body can build, maintain, and repair its own tissues, and it is our job to provide the raw nutritional material, and keep our internal environment free of the things that get in the way.

Of course the only option for treatment of disease is from the only school of medicine *legally qualified* to "treat" a "disease." But we're not taught about the option of supporting the body's ability to heal itself. The mainstream medical world talks nothing of the body's ability to heal itself. Here's more from Healthline.com:

> Allopathic medicine is also called allopathy. It's a health system in which medical doctors, nurses, pharmacists, and other healthcare professionals are licensed to practice and treat symptoms and diseases.

> Treatment is done with:
> - medication
> - surgery
> - radiation
> - other therapies and procedures

On the other side of the fence are the fields that believe the body can heal itself, given the right ingredients and environment. The body grew itself, all by itself. The body can produce all of it's own hormones, neurotransmitters, enzymes, and so on. It produces its own stem cells. It can regulate its own temperature, organs, blood nutrient levels, and so on.

The holistic side of the fence believes that all pharmaceutical interventions are harmful, even when some may be entirely necessary, particularly in the case of infections. But even in emergencies, we do not believe that drugs are a "cure", unless the "disease" was caused directly by an infection, which is killed by a drug and thus cured.

Gratefully, doctors don't talk much about cures, so there is not much argument about the actual reversal of disease. They manage diseases, and it's quite literally not their job to cure them. When we aim to restore health and eliminate all signs of a disease, we are therefore not competing with doctors, as their aim is to manage the symptoms, not eliminate them.

We would prefer our customers not to have diseases or symptoms or concerns. We would prefer to help them get out of pain, but it is not us doing the work. It is with basic, mostly forgotten, often forbidden nutritional strategies that are as old as humanity.

The only thing truly preventing the average person from attaining good health is the barrier to information in the medical marketplace. The language around disease dictates the way we respond to disease. The monopoly in this marketplace is held by a profession that does not believe the body can heal itself. Due to this monopoly in the public image of "healthcare", the average person simply does not know about the other options.

These paragraphs serve as the disclaimer, that we are not really arguing the necessity of some of the most common medical interventions. Some surgeries are necessary. Many are not. Antibiotics save lives, and they are also over prescribed and can cause serious long term damage to those patients.

Some tests could be useful, but in practice, we don't really need tests. We don't need to see blood work, and in fact most people who come to us with "diseases" tell us that their blood is "fine" according to their doctors. They come to us with health problems and previous diagnosis of diseases, but their blood is fine. So the charts don't help us that much anyway. These days, we don't even see our customers in real life in most cases, since we operate primarily online. We don't need to touch them or take their temperature. We just need to give them advice that actually works.

2. Birth Defects.

Let's start with the easy "diseases." We are told that birth defects are diseases. But in our holistic understanding, all birth defects are environmental. Something was missing in the development process, or something harmful interfered with the process.

Which part of this is a lack of ease? This is a mechanical issue. Someone steps away from the assembly line, and a part does not make it onto the car.

The medical profession that is responsible for birthing children in the "developed world" are allopathic MDs. It is worth mentioning that nutrition is not a required course in the study of becoming an allopathic professional. Mainstream medicine seems to believe that nutrition is overrated, or at least that we can "get everything we need by eating all the food groups."

We have a lengthy explanation as to why it is not true that "we can get everything we need by eating all the food groups." But it is simpler to talk about animals as the starting point.

Thankfully, it is not a legal issue to talk about *preventing* birth defects in animals. It is standard business to maintain flocks, herds, or colonies of animals without birth defects.

Notice that the word "cure" here is not relevant. Part of my reasoning for calling these diseases "fake", is *not* that they don't occur – birth defects are "real", they do occur – but that this language doesn't make sense. You don't "catch" a birth defect. The cause is multi-dimensional, as are most of the topics we will cover. But even if the cause is understood, in the case of birth defects there is no "cure."

So how can we "run for a cure" if the only option in birth defects is to prevent them or put up with them once they have occurred? Most birth defects can't be reversed after they've already happened. You can see how this thinking of diseases and cures is entirely mis-leading by glancing at a list of only a few birth defects:

- type 1 diabetes[i]
- Down's syndrome
- heart defects
- cystic fibrosis
- cleft lips, cleft palate
- hernias
- limb defects
- sickle cell anemia/thalassemia[ii]

Each of these are understood and prevented in every animal in domestic care. In humans, most of these are thought of as unique to humans and transmitted through genetics. Usually they have different names in animals than in humans. Farmers don't need to know most of the names because they will probably never have to deal with them, simply by following regular nutritional protocols by the book.

For example. Muscular dystrophy in humans is referred to as a disease. A disease in need of a cure. MedicalNewsToday.com said in 2020 the average life expectancy of a muscular dystrophy patient nowadays is 26 years old. They say plainly, "there is no cure." Fundraising efforts have continued for decades. New treatments are actively being tested, they say.

In animals this problem is known as white muscle disease. It is caused by a selenium deficiency. Even though the word "disease" is part of the name, there is no confusion because animal diseases do not legally require a "licensed medical practitioner" to deal with them. The prevention and reversal of white muscle disease is taught to farmers, both in agricultural school and at the feed store. Selenium is usually given by injection into pregnant livestock.

Feeds are regularly fortified with the mineral selenium, and its co-factors,[1] particularly iodine. Most of the topsoil on Earth is barren of selenium.

I am neither a farmer nor a veterinarian, but this is common knowledge across the world. For some reason we believe all animals have similar pathogenesis (development of disease), and we give common disease names across the animal kingdom. So, in every other large animal you can name, muscular dystrophy is called white muscle disease, and is prevented with the same protocol. With humans it is a different name and so we can be forgiven for missing the connection. Alas, we are animals. Our nutritional requirements are roughly the same as every other animal, and we all get the same diseases from the same nutritional deficiencies, however we choose to name them.

It could be a very long list. But suffice to say, we, meaning humanity, have "cured" all of these birth defect problems in animals, by prevention. Animal husbandry is as old as society, as far as we know. All industries involving animals have eliminated all birth defects. All animals. All birth defects.

It also has nothing to do with inbreeding. It is standard practice to inbreed practically every animal you can think of without a problem. In most cases of domestic breeds, particularly in the pet industry, inbreeding has occurred for dozens of generations. No birth defects, except in the case of born runts or stillborns.

Healthy animals often have large litters, or many eggs. It is not necessarily a sign of a problem with the mother to have a runt or two. The rest of her babies should be in "perfect" condition.

Perfect is a word you don't see too often in medical reference to a human. But in the animal industries, "perfect" means "normal." It is perfectly normal to have a healthy litter from a healthy mother, and have a runt or a stillborn in the batch. Or an egg with nothing in it. It happens.

---

1 A cofactor is a nutrient that is required for the other nutrient to function properly. For example, iron and copper are direct cofactors, and thus a deficiency of copper can look like symptoms of iron deficiency.

Goats commonly have twins, and every farmer knows that one just might not make it. One is stronger from the start. In the wild, one has a real chance. Often the mother abandons the runt. Sometimes its not even a clear runt. It is very common to have one of the twins rejected, especially in young mothers. Farmers are used to bottle feeding the rejects. Sometimes the mother kills it on purpose. Infanticide saves important resources in the wild.

Runts are not always birth defects. The mothers can be prize-winning animals that achieve their proper longevity and never experience illness or infection. Inbred for generations. Given the proper nutritional environment, generational perfection is basically guaranteed. Anyone can learn to be a farmer and do this.

Western medicine does not apply this to humans. My mentor, Dr. Joel Wallach, has sued the Food and Drug Administration (FDA) multiple times successfully, often in reference to birth defects and essential nutrients. As a veterinarian before becoming a licensed medical practitioner on humans, he knew that much human suffering was already eliminated in animals long ago, especially birth defects. That's in animal husbandry 101. He and others have secured several "qualified health claims" from the FDA, and mandates to include these nutrients in prenatal formulas and baby foods.

In the case of many birth defects, if the nutrient was not present near the beginning of the pregnancy, the defect has already occurred. It is these early mistakes that can lead to larger problems in development. So nutritional deficiencies early in pregnancy are not addressed by taking prenatal formulas or baby foods.

The nutrients needed to be present before the woman would have a chance to know they are pregnant. Most women don't start taking prenatal formulas until they've missed two periods. That is too late for much of the list of birth defects to be rectified.

So, most birth defects cannot be cured after the animal or human is born, because they have already happened. The glass is broken. The leg isn't there, the mouth isn't big enough to fit all of the teeth, the gland isn't equipped to do it's job, the brain is underdeveloped, whatever it is.

Calling a birth defect a "disease" completely misses the cause of the problem. The medical profession has no explanation for the cause of much of the list above. I don't mean that they have an explanation that we disagree with – there's lots of those – I mean they honestly don't know. The name of the disease has not helped us, and calling it a disease has not helped us.

When something is labeled a disease it falls under the jurisdiction of the allopathic medical profession. This profession has no clear understanding of the cause, prevention, or "cure" of this category. They do not claim to.

No birth defect will ever be "cured." The language doesn't even make sense. In recent years sudden infant death syndrome has decreased dramatically in America. This decline coincides with the FDA mandate, secured by Dr. Wallach, to include selenium in baby formulas. Part of the work used to secure the claim is the connection between selenium deficiency and sudden infant death syndrome.[iii]

When this was announced in various state and national newspapers, most of them didn't use the word "cure", to my knowledge. They didn't know why, but the occurrence of sudden infant death syndrome was just disappearing.

We'd like to see more diseases "disappear." They will disappear long before they are called "cured" by the allopathic medical world. Even when an individual patient has been "in remission" from a disease for decades, the patient is not declared cured.

Really, we don't even have a framework to begin saying anything has been cured. We can eliminate symptoms. They can vanish. People can change their lifestyles, they can consume more nutrients, they can appear by all measures to be perfectly healthy after being diagnosed with a disease, but they can never legally be declared "cured." You would think that "cure" and "eliminated" are the same. Apparently not.

Selenium is just one of the essential minerals. Minerals are the largest category of essential nutrients. They're arguably the most important category, because all of the degenerative diseases are mineral deficiency diseases.[iv] In our belief, there are at least 59 other essential minerals, and 30 other distinct nutrients that are essential to the proper "structure and function" of our body. We need them to develop properly, to function properly, and to repair ourselves.

If certain nutrients are missing during development, a specific birth defect will be present. If many are missing, the child can be born with several "diseases", or the pregnancy is miscarried. If those same nutrients are missing later in life, a "disease" is the result. One of the reasons that essential nutrients are called "essential" is because without them, we get a "disease."

Medical doctors recognize this, by the way. They just have a shorter list of essential nutrients, they believe you need less of them than we believe, and they think you can get these nutrients by eating all the food groups.

Medical doctors also recognize several birth defects as nutrient deficiencies, especially as more and more such claims are filed against the FDA. But their only advice is to use the prenatal formulas once a woman is pregnant. Again, this is too late to prevent much of the list.

As far as I can tell, the only reason the medical profession is able to convey the idea that birth defects are in fact diseases at all, is their theory that many of these problems are "transmitted" genetically.

I have said that part of my problem in calling something a disease, is the implication that you can "catch" it. In reality, most disease is a name for a collection of symptoms. The reason there are so many disease names, is that there are so many different symptoms, and an even larger number of potential combinations of symptoms. If a person has all the signs of a disease, but also has other symptoms, often it is named a new disease. This adds to the confusion.

So, by the logic of the medical profession, relying on the theory that birth defects are transmitted genetically, they are able to call it a disease and call for a cure. And research money. And pharmaceutical intervention.

Well, in animals none of this is considered genetic. If an animal is born with a defect, it is considered the fault of the farmer or zoo keeper or pet shop owner. If your snakes are born with crooked spines, it is your fault. If they can't make it out of the egg because their egg tooth hasn't developed, it is your fault for failing to provide them enough minerals to do so. It was not transmitted from mother to baby. It was a problem on the conveyor belt.

Except in humans, apparently.

The mainstream medical world not only believes that most or all birth defects are "genetically transmitted", they also believe many other types of problems are caused by your genetics as well. Genes don't change quickly, yet disease frequency absolutely does. They say that over a third of the American population currently has diabetes or prediabetes, and this surging prevalence is less than a hundred years old.

Our genes haven't changed much, or at all, in the last hundred years, but our lifestyles and nutrient availability in our food supply most certainly has. Often MDs will say "this disease has a 20 or 40 or 80% connection to genetics", and I believe that all of these numbers are pure nonsense. All of the common diseases you or someone you know is dealing with, have been prevented and eliminated in animals. They have absolutely nothing to do with genetics, and everything to do with nutrients and the environment.

In all this talk of fake, or mislabeled, or misleading "diseases", you will find no evidence of any disease that is genetically transmitted. Every disease we can name, we have the corresponding disease in animals already mapped out, and we have eliminated every single one of them in standard practice.

It is only by tragic ignorance or misunderstanding that we treat ourselves, and the way we think about our own diseases, differently from animals. Most of us never get a chance to stop and wonder why we are the only species that can get a disease via genetics.

3. Sexually Transmitted Diseases.

When I was a kid, people came by our school and gave us a seminar about sexually transmitted diseases. We were told that sex could lead to disease. Scary.

I will deal with AIDS and the related "H viruses" separately later in the book. The rest of the "STDs" were unceremoniously renamed to "sexually transmitted infections", or STIs. They just changed the letter.

Renaming is common. But this one is appreciated. Many adults today still give me a puzzled look when I tell them: "there are no sexually transmitted diseases."

An infection is not a disease in the sense of the rest of the problems in this book. An infection is different from osteoporosis or diabetes or cancer. The only reason we call all of these things diseases is so they can be legally treated by the allopathic profession.

One of my problems with calling so many things "diseases", is the common definition is lost. An infection and a birth defect are wildly different things. The body falling apart is different from catching a bacterial infection. Giving birth is much different than saving an accident victim. But these are all spoken of together in one bundle primarily because one profession has claimed responsibility for the whole lot.

How are we to know the difference between important types of health problems, if we call them all the same thing? What if we called all the colors "blue?" Hey could you hand me the blue? No, the other blue!

Would you bring your car to a guy who spent most of his time fixing pianos and refurbishing old furniture? It's all the same thing right?

We can "catch" an infection. And we can also, legally, cure an infection. Syphilis is cured with penicillin. This is legal language. It is the correct terminology.

Notice that the word "cure" is entirely appropriate in this situation. A bug, in this case *Treponema pallidum*, is killed by penicillin. The problem has a direct observable cause, and once the bug is killed, the problem is completely eliminated. It will not recur unless re-exposed. A cancer patient without symptoms is forever in remission, but if you had a sexually transmitted infection, it was cured by an antibiotic.

All of the STIs are indeed infections, which is why it is good that they renamed them. Unfortunately, the overall language of disease still obfuscates the truth. Through the control of language, the treatment is also controlled. I believe that one of the many reasons STIs are promoted so heavily, (or, at least they used to be), is that they are one of the only things that give MDs their ability to claim they are the only legitimate practitioners of medicine. "We cured syphilis! Trust us with everything else."

The branch of pharmaceuticals known as anti-biotics have their purpose defined in the name. They kill biotics. A biological agent infects a body, and we know a corresponding chemical that neutralizes that bug in many cases.

These infections are not as common as you would think. I hardly ever come across anyone claiming to have an STI. We are almost never asked about it. The younger generations today do not seem worried about them. My parents' generation wasn't really worried about them in the first place. My age group was given the full scare treatment as kids, but the hype has largely died down about it.

More unfortunately, the medical profession over time has used their successes in curing infections as justification for pursuing pharmaceutical intervention in other, non-infectious diseases. This is how we get disease management with pharmaceutical drugs. And it was never justified. Infections are not like most diseases. Antibiotic treatment is not long term, and success is measurable and observable. This does not apply to any other diseases on our list.

The one category that mainstream medicine *can* cure, are not even called diseases anymore.

It is worth mentioning that syphilis was officially cured in 1943. Aside from infections, there has not been a single disease cured by drugs, surgery, or any other mainstream western treatment.

We can catch infections via sex. We can also catch an infection by scraping our knee on the pavement, or by improper tattoo aftercare. But these are not diseases. Your mother doesn't tell you to clean out your cut "or you'll get a disease!"

Antibacterial soap comes in many forms. We would recommend using natural soaps that you can understand the ingredients of, but even a cheap chemical antibacterial soap will prevent most wounds from becoming infected. The potential for infection is always present. All a person has to do to decrease their chances of getting an infection, is to keep their wounds clean.[v]

Internal infections I believe are very similar. I have no evidence that sexually transmitted infections are different from wound infections, in the sense that, it doesn't matter where on Earth you are, if you fail to keep your wounds clean, they will become infected.

Our world is awash with bacteria and viruses and micro organisms of endless variety. It is commonly said that around 90% of our body cells are bacteria, viruses, and protozoa, which are tiny animals. We have all kinds of "bad" microorganisms in our bodies, even when we are healthy, such as *Escherichia coli*, and candida yeasts like *Candida albicans*. I believe the potential for internal infection is the same as external infection. If we fail to keep our internal environment clean, we provide the environment for bad bacteria to thrive.

Here I am talking about the internal environment of the digestive system. We will cover this in more detail later, as it applies to many common infections such as ear, sinus, and urinary tract, as well as a proclivity to fungal infections and more.

But the other "internal" environment in the case of sexually transmitted infections, is the cavities of the sex organs themselves. It is no wonder that STIs are more common in women than men. More dark, damp space for bacteria to thrive if it is not washed thoroughly, especially after sex. I believe that a majority of the cases I have seen could have been prevented just by showering after sex, instead of falling asleep. If a tattoo is infected, it could have been prevented with hygiene.

This does not mean that you are unhygenic if you ever got an STI. A person can be perfectly clean all day, get their orifices dirty, fall asleep and wake up with an infection.

This is not proven. But it is my observation with my handful of cases that each person I have seen experiencing an STI, has other symptoms of an internal digestive environment that is off. I just have not seen an otherwise perfectly healthy person with an STI. In my theory, a person can still have a one-off unclean night, and have themselves a problem, even if they eat well, but they are far more likely to experience any type of infection if they have an internal environment that promotes the growth of bad bacteria, fungus, and so on.

Some people call this "terrain theory." This implies that the infection is not out there trying to get us. The theory is that we are always in a sea of bacteria and viruses. We do not seem to have a problem with them as long as our body is healthy and clean.

In any case, if any of us catches an STI, there is an antibiotic ready for us. There are also many natural herbal alternatives. STIs often aren't that serious, and many people can rid themselves of symptoms simply by consuming cranberry extract or taking a common anti-microbial tincture such as oil of oregano or olive leaf extract.

4. Bone & Joint Diseases.

This is one of the largest categories of disease. There are currently over 200 diseases listed in the *Physicians' Desk Reference* with the same nutritional deficiency root. Many of these are the bone and joint diseases themselves, but it is worth seeing a short list of the types of problems in this category:

- ankylosing spondylitis
- arthritis
- back pain
- Bell's palsy
- bone fractures
- bone spurs
- brittle fingernails
- calcium deposits
- cartilage damage
- cognitive impairment
- delusions
- depression
- Dowager's hump
- elevated blood calcium
- eczema
- high/low blood pressure
- hyperactivity
- hyperparathyroidism
- insomnia
- irritability
- joint pain
- kidney stones
- limb numbness
- muscle cramps
- nervousness
- neuromuscular excitability
- osteofibrosis
- osteomalacia
- osteoporosis
- palpitations
- panic attacks
- paresthesia
- periodontal disease
- pica (munchies)
- prolonged clotting time
- receding gums
- restless legs

- retarded growth
- rickets
- sciatica
- spasms/twitches
- spinal stenosis

- tetany
- tinnitus
- tooth decay
- vertigo

Not a fun list. Many of these problems have other nutrient deficiencies involved. These really are true diseases in the sense of a lack of health. None of these are caught and cured like the infectious diseases (there is one exception we will get to), and like birth defects, the mainstream medical world has no official idea what causes, prevents, or "cures" any of them.

There is more than one reason I called this book *Fake Diseases*. This category of disease is very real, very unpleasant, and very expensive. But this group of problems were eliminated a thousand years ago in Chinese agricultural history. It was rediscovered in Europe centuries ago as well. And in the 20th century it was biochemically mapped the modern way and addressed nutritionally, with complete success. We figured it out in animals, it just has not been applied to humans by the allopathic profession, and so we don't hear much about it.

You might have noticed that the only medical professionals you have probably ever seen on television, film, or the media in general, were allopathic doctors, nurses, pharmacists, and scientists. There are no dramas about the holistic world that I know of. We are subliminally educated to see disease in the allopathic view partially because it is the only one we are exposed to in our modern lives.

Sometimes we hear of the quacks with the dark glass bottles of snake oil. Not many people are persuaded to look into holistic protocols with this type of a widespread mainstream opinion about them. Likely the witty protagonist doctor on the TV, between heroically saving lives, will find screen time to bash the quacks at least once each episode. Likely the late night pundit will find time as well. As will the newscaster. Completely coincidental.

The reason I call this category of disease "fake", is because this seems like a scam. Why have 200 things we call a disease, when we have we have eliminated these in livestock a thousand years ago in ancient times, again in medieval times, and again in modern times?

Modern medicine does not cure anything on the list. Dog food prevents all of it. Doctors manage the symptoms with drugs or surgery or psychiatry, indefinitely. Dogs don't have health insurance.[vi] Many honest physicians refuse to recommend patients for joint replacement surgeries they know to be useless, but their toolkit still does not have much else besides pharmaceutical painkillers and anti-inflammatory drugs.

Calling something a disease legally puts it in the umbrella of allopathic medicine. It doesn't matter if illiterate farmers figured this out a thousand years ago. In humans, a disease must be managed by a licensed medical practitioner – unless you take things into your own hands.

You are legally allowed to treat yourself, we're just not allowed to treat you. And you can represent yourself in court, or hire a professional and take their advice. Or take advice from a guy on the street or internet. As we go on, you can see how all of this legal language makes less and less sense when applied to health problems. It only makes sense when we realize it was designed to define medical practice itself.

Each of the problems in the bone and joint category is due to deficiency of the nutrient group that makes up bones. As a shorthand, we can refer to it as "the calcium family." Sometimes we might even just say calcium. But it is the entire web of nutrients around this important mineral that is also necessary for the proper structure and function of our body.

Structure in this case is literal. Our bones are made of stuff that we need more of. Joints are made of the same stuff, more or less. And this mineral and its cofactor friends are also required for several "functions" in the body. Notice the behavioral problems in the list above. And the soft-tissue problems such as eczema and periodontal disease. Muscles are also governed by this same nutrient group. Calcium is required for every muscle contraction, magnesium for every muscle relaxation. These nutrients need to be in balance, along with their many cofactors, or there will be a muscle problem, which also appear on the list above.

If one nutrient, or nutrient group is needed for a variety of functions in the body – in this case the same mineral responsible for many "functions" is also a building material for the structure itself, as if a brick building were also lighted and heated by brick – then a deficiency in that nutrient can lead to a variety of problems.

We cannot always predict which symptoms will occur with a deficiency in the calcium group, since the body has to decide where to use it. You may have tooth decay but not back pain. You may have the whole list. The tree can fall in many directions.

We like to refer to "the wisdom of the body." The body is intelligent, we say. Smarter than our doctor, I might say. But intelligence can only go so far. If an intelligent body has to choose between functions because it has a lack of resources, the result is still going to be a problem. A professional building crew will have a problem if they are short on essential materials. A brand new car will not start without a spark plug, and it will preform poorly if the oil is not changed and other fluids are not topped up.

When minerals are used in functions in the body, rather than structure, it is useful to think of them as spark plugs. They activate things. They allow other processes to happen. Reactions to happen and transmitters to fire, and so on.

It is likely that someone with arthritis will also have other symptoms they recognize on the list at the start of this chapter. By addressing the underlying deficiencies involved in arthritis, they should find improvement in the other problems as well, because the same material is used as spark plugs for numerous functions, as well as building material for the bones and joints themselves, as well as gums and teeth and other soft tissues.

There is an age old saying in the holistic world: "Like treats like." This phrase is technically illegal if taken literally. The principle comes from what is known as the "theory of signatures." A walnut looks like a brain and thus was thought to "support and promote maintenance and repair of healthy brains." We do now know that walnuts and other such brainy foods are in fact high in the fat soluble nutrients required for optimal brain function. These are essential nutrients for many functions in the body, particularly in the brain.

The theory can be extended to red being good for blood, and of course, our point here, bones and joints being good for bones and joints.

Yes, we eliminated this list of diseases and symptoms in animals a thousand years ago, by adding ground bones and joints to livestock feeds. In the field, cows, horses, pigs, sheep, and goats will all opportunistically forage on small animals. Yes, horses and cows will eat small snakes, birds, rodents, eggs, and they will likely chew on any bones that happen to be in the fields. They do this instinctively.

If an animal is mineral deficient (any mineral, but this calcium group in particular), this "pica" behavior will become stronger. They will chew on the wood of the barns or fences, the handles of tools, and each others' horns and even hoofs. Typically this behavior can be stopped by giving them bone meal and/or a salt block, also called a salt lick. The block contains a spread of trace minerals and should stop the "cribbing", which is the gnawing chewing craving symptom of "pica."

This is the wisdom of the body. It requires minerals to maintain and repair its structure and function. It asks for these in the form of a craving. If the nutrients are not provided, the body will continue to be hungry. It will continue to crib. Most people just make the mistake of feeding the body *food*, rather than feeding it the missing nutrients. This problem is not helped by a medical profession that tells the public we "can get everything we need by eating the food groups," and "those people selling calcium supplements are quacks."

I mentioned salt and calcium together because they are important cofactors, and this is why I believe they can both be effective in eliminating the cribbing in animals, and in humans.

Bone and joint problems are a result of a lack of bones and joints, quite literally. Human populations in the wild use most of every animal they catch, including the bones. In many cases the bones can be eaten directly from a cooked bird or fish or small animal. Bigger bones are often ground into a flour that is added into pretty much every type of dish you could name."[2] Other bones are boiled in soups or stocks. The natural human consumes bones in some form essentially every day.

These diseases are fake because they are called diseases just so they fall under the jurisdiction of allopathic medicine. If these problems were called what they are literally: "symptoms of multiple nutrient deficiencies", I imagine it would be very difficult to persuade a regular citizen to take pharmaceutical drugs with side effects and no promise of improvement and no cure word available. It would be more difficult to persuade a customer to have their knees replaced if it were called a nutrient deficiency.

This is because deficiencies can be corrected. I hope that is obvious. It is not obvious to allopathic professionals. I have actually been called a liar by allopathic professionals for claiming that cartilage could be regrown. I didn't know it was a controversial claim. It is an observable occurrence.

Remember that a disease is a name for a group of symptoms. If the symptoms are a result of a nutrient deficiency, then so are the diseases named after them. If a deficiency can be corrected, then the symptoms can "disappear." This is not a miracle. This is farming.

This is also not a cure. Again we find that cure is not even an appropriate word here. The word "disease" is misleading because of this.

Let's now cover the exception, rheumatoid arthritis. This view on rheumatoid arthritis is not accepted in the mainstream medical community, and it is also not widely accepted in the alternative community. There is no agreement on what causes it, but you don't need scientific consensus to do something about it yourself.

We have an explanation that is very hard to find if you just searched "rheumatoid." You'll first find it being referred to as an "autoimmune" disease. We will cover autoimmune problems later.

---

2   "Fee-fi-fo-fum

   I smell the blood of an Englishman.

   Be he alive or be he dead

   I'll grind his **bones** to make my **bread**."

- Jack and the Beanstock

In our view, the rheumatoid component of the problem is an infection with a bacteria called *mycoplasma*.

The infection causes damage. The proper response from a body when it is experiencing damage, is to "inflame." This brings blood and resources to the area. Pain signifies the desire for the body to keep you from further damaging the area. This particular bug is also known to cause respiratory infections and this is probably why it is thought to be an autoimmune problem.

In this case, the bug must be killed. As an alternative practitioner, I cannot prescribe pharmaceuticals. Dr. Wallach recommends the antibiotic minocycline.[vii] Of course, you would have to talk to a licensed medical practitioner about this. They probably won't believe you. But if you have been suffering, and nothing else has worked, it is probably not that hard to persuade them to give this a supervised try.

There are natural antimicrobial compounds and products that can be effective if used seriously and in conjunction with a food protocol. But the pharmaceutical antibiotic is much more reliable.

Once the bug is killed the tissues need to be rebuilt just like any other bone or joint degeneration. It needs more of the stuff it is made of in order to rebuild itself. This book is not going to go into specific detail on products, doses, or diets. This is the base information, and I encourage you to contact us or whoever gave you this book, to talk more specifically about what might be best for you. Our contact information is at the back of the book.

5. Blood Sugar Diseases.

Now things get a bit more complicated.

We saw type 1 diabetes listed as a birth defect. We call it an "inborn error of metabolism", in this case affecting the pancreatic cells that produce insulin, "beta cells." Birth defects can be prevented, but not always reversed. People born with any birth defect also tend to have other health problems. Maybe immune problems, weight problems, skin, digestion, brain fog, migraines, back pain. Just like any other person on the street, a type 1 diabetic or a cystic fibrosis patient can also have other common complaints, or even another disease.

Blood sugar is one of the problems that you can have with any other disease. The type 1 will probably need synthetic insulin for the rest of their lives, since they are not producing enough on their own.[3] But other markers of health can still improve by correcting the diet, and by consuming all of the essential nutrients.

The blood is the transport system of the body. It transports nutrients around and delivers them to cells throughout the body. It transports oxygen from the lungs, and nutrients from the digestive

---

3 Many people report that they were diagnosed as T1 and no longer need insulin after changing their diet and/or adding proper supplements. Our assumption is that they were misdiagnosed and were in fact type 2 diabetics, which is reversible.

system. The veins in our body get smaller and smaller until they reach literally every other cell in our body. It is quite amazing. Everything is connected to the blood.

Whatever food we eat, the body turns it into sugar (glucose) and feeds it to our cells. Sugar is essential, and it is not itself the enemy, but we don't need to consume it directly. We can convert fat and protein, as well as carbs, into sugar to feed the cells.

We need nutrients to process sugar. We need nutrients to digest anything. Two of the key minerals involved in healthy blood sugar, chromium and vanadium, have at least 23 other direct nutrient cofactors. Really, we would connect it all to the cake recipe of the 90 essential nutrients.

These two key nutrients are needed to process sugar. They are needed for "healthy blood sugar." We know this from the animal industries, which eliminated all blood sugar related problems officially in the 1950s.

This information was actually widely known at some times, due to media publicity. Evidently many of the listeners who ran out and started buying chromium and vanadium, did not avoid the modern plagues of diabetes and related problems. This is because of the 88 other nutrients involved in a "healthy body", and the many other factors that can contribute stress on the system.

So, we need at least two nutrients to process sugar, and those two are largely deficient in the food supply, soils, and home supplement cabinets. That's one part of the problem.

The next part of the problem is the amount of sugar we actually eat. If we need 1 unit of x nutrient to process 1 unit of sugar, we are going to need much more of x nutrient if we greatly increase our average consumption of sugar.

We consume much more sugar today than we did a hundred or two hundred years ago. I have seen many estimates of exactly how much more we consume, ranging from twice as much to 300 times as much, but since there are different criteria involved (processed and "natural" sugars are sometimes calculated differently), and since not everyone eats the same way, I will avoid pinning down a number. The point is that we consume more than we used to. We're claiming that we already had a nutrient deficiency problem going on a hundred years ago, but then we increased our need for that nutrient, on average, by however many times more sugar we consume. So we need 2-300 times more of those nutrients, and their cofactors, for the body to be able to process the sugar we consume.

Here is a list of potential symptoms or diseases related to blood sugar problems:

- anxiety
- adrenal failure/chronic fatigue
- bed wetting
- cardiovascular disease
- depression
- diabetes
- elevated cholesterol & triglycerides (hypercholesterolemia)
- fainting
- hyperactivity
- hypoglycemia (low blood sugar)
- infertility
- learning disabilities
- migraine headaches
- moodiness
- narcolepsy
- night sweats/night teeth grinding
- obesity
- peripheral neuropathy
- retarded growth
- short lifespan

You might have noticed that retarded growth was also on the calcium deficiency list. As all 90 essential nutrients overlap, there is also overlap on the symptoms and disease lists of each deficiency.

Elevated blood cholesterol and triglycerides are likely the first sign of a blood sugar problem. The cellular explanation is quite complicated. The point is, anyone with a blood sugar problem, or diabetes, will most likely also have anxiety issues, chronic fatigue, high blood cholesterol, and ultimately a reduced lifespan.

This is because the blood is the most important thing in the body. These warning signs like high cholesterol signify a major problem in the body. Circulation problems are inevitable if this continues, as cholesterol clogs up the blood, making it harder to circulate. Healthy blood sugar is extremely important to a healthy body and a happy life. Blood sugar fluctuations, in our view, are given several behavioral disease names you will recognize:

- ADD/ADHD
- bipolar disorder
- seasonal affective disorder
- mood disorders generally
- autism and other behavioral disorders

In the next chapter we are going to cover digestion diseases, but it is worth laying some groundwork here. Any digestive problem, whatever it is caused by, can cause a blood sugar problem. A nutrient deficiency can cause a blood sugar problem, but a digestive problem can *cause the deficiency*. A digestive problem can interfere with nutrient absorption, in the end causing a blood sugar problem.

Once there is a blood sugar problem, as we know, one of the first consequences is elevated cholesterol. One of the consequences of this is a compromised circulatory system.

So how to have healthy blood sugar? Other than providing the body with the essential nutrients for the job, it is very wise of us to limit processed sugar to an absolute minimum.

Often we are asked if it is okay to replace, say, sugar in coffee with honey or syrup. I usually say that this is largely more habitual, or an actual addiction to sugar, than any sort of necessity. Quantity is the primary problem. You cannot escape sugar, because the body will turn all of your food into sugar to feed the cells, but you can limit the excess of sugar entering the system.

Honey and syrup were prized and difficult to obtain luxuries in the wild environment. They are still luxuries and should be limited. Completely abstaining from all powder or liquid sugar for around two weeks is usually enough to break the cravings and the habit. Fruit or dried fruit is fine, but if you find yourself gorging on it then you can see there is a problem.

Cut the body off from this addiction. We recommend replacing carbs in general and sugar in particular with various fats, proteins, and plant material in the diet. A sugar craving can often be stopped by eating protein instead, or by consuming minerals. Even a glass of salty water can often stop a sugar craving.

People with diabetes or who are alcoholics should of course reduce the intake of sugar and alcohol, but if you find yourself lightheaded or dizzy (low blood sugar), it is wise to eat something. Dried fruit will bring your blood sugar up quickly in a much healthier way than a candy bar or beer.

The last major component to healthy blood sugar is digestion, which will be covered in the next chapter. But it is worth wrapping up blood sugar into the fake disease conversation by recapping that, type 1 diabetes is a birth defect, and all birth defects are preventable, not "cure"able, and so in my opinion it should not rightly be called a disease. If it can be cured with treatment then it is fine to classify it in responsibility to licensed professionals who handle treatment. But we can't reverse birth defects that have already happened, at least not this particular one.

The best we can do to prevent type 1 from occurring is to support a healthy pregnancy, by encouraging women to consume all 90 essential nutrients *before and during* pregnancy, and avoiding the foods that get in the way of absorbing nutrients. People are still walking for the cure for type 1 diabetes, but if they called it what they would in animals, "a nutrient deficiency in embryo", then they could clearly see the real solution: prevention.

All of those behavioral problems don't seem rightly described as "diseases" either. Ten years ago I was under the impression that an autistic child likely had visible developmental problems as well, sort of like Asperger's syndrome. Now any kid with a behavioral problem (likely just a blood sugar problem), can be called "diseased."

This is not logical or fair. A blood sugar problem does not need to be managed with pharmaceutical drugs, none of which are designed to "cure" the problem, none of which could possibly cure the problem because the problem is caused by nutrient deficiencies and the wrong foods.

These things are called diseases so they can be treated by licensed allopathic medical professionals. It's big business, to put it lightly. Diabetes has been called the most expensive disease in recent years, before 2020 hit of course.

Blood sugar related behavioral problems are not "diseases." The body can achieve healthy blood sugar quite quickly. Type 2 diabetics regularly get off their medication, with or without the supervision or support of the allopathic medical doctor who put them on their drug program.

In the case of type 2 diabetes itself, as well as all the behavioral blood sugar problems, the difference between reversal and a cure is important. We don't catch diabetes or autism. Blood sugar is constantly in flux. If it is low, you might be moody. You might eat something and get a spike and then get tired. This can happen in minutes. And the body can achieve healthy blood sugar quickly as well. This can be measured by the regular mainstream medical world, and of course you can measure your own blood sugar any time you want with test strips from a pharmacy.

Knowing all of this, I hope you can understand the frustration I have felt every time I see fundraisers to raise money for pharmaceutical research on these problems. The allopathic way is to interfere chemically with processes in the body. Most types of drugs are named by the way they interfere with something in the body. Anti-inflammatory drugs interfere with inflammation. Inflammation is a natural response to a damaged tissue or pathogen threat. A drug that blocks pain also blocks the signal our body is telling us to go easy on that area or address it.

To me, any problem that we call a disease, but is regularly prevented or even reversed in animals, and also widely reversed in humans, just should not be called a disease. That is false advertising. Things are called diseases so they can be treated by allopathic doctors, nurses, surgeons, and pharmacists.

These professions do not claim to have a cure for these diseases, they only have pharmaceutical management, or cutting out parts or replacing them. If we continue to think of behavior problems, or blood sugar problems, in terms of disease, we will continue to believe that these should be "treated", of course by the only profession legally entitled to "treat" any diseases.

Since it's called a disease, we run to a doctor. If we understand it as a process having to do with food, nutrients, and digestion, it is much easier to deal with – yourself. I have gone into much more detail about blood sugar and what to do about it in my book *Everything You Should Know About Healthy Blood Sugar*. The subtitle of that book is *Simple Strategies to Conquer Almost Any Health Problem*, because blood sugar problems are connected to most of the things that people come to us about, and also because implementing strategies to achieve healthy blood sugar will probably alleviate most other problems a person could have.

Let's return to syphilis for a moment, because we are at the core of the whole *Fake Diseases* theory.

Syphilis is a disease, correctly termed.

Because diseases should be treated by medical professionals: doctors, nurses, and pharmacists. Surgeries and surgeons are necessary when a person is hit by a car, shot with a bullet, and also in removing growths in the body and other potential emergency interventions. This in my opinion should be the professional boundary of the allopathic profession.

If you have syphilis, you should absolutely go to a medical doctor.

The treatment is penicillin.

It is cured, you pay, or insurance pays, and the deal is done.

But blood sugar problems do not follow this logical route. Blood sugar problems do not require medicine. They do not require medical or surgical or pharmaceutical intervention.

Type 1 diabetes would seem to be an exception here. It does require management with insulin. Insulin is a hormone. It is packaged and prescribed by the medical profession, but it is not a drug, technically. It's called a drug because it's used to manage a "disease." This one example of a birth defect being helped with a synthetic hormone gives justification for other diseases to be "managed" with totally different types of drugs.

This also applies to some other drugs and cancer treatments. Lithium is known as a drug. In our field, we know it as an essential mineral, and we know it to be important for overall mental health. A mineral is a nutrient, and so it cannot be patented. But they can add a bunch of other ingredients and patent that.

I still don't think it's correct to call type 1 diabetes a disease for this reason. It does not require a licensed practitioner to dispense a synthetic hormone. They sell vitamin D at the grocery store, an important and essential hormone. Even if a professional needed to be involved, they only need to be diagnosed once. The treatment is the same for the rest of their life: synthetic insulin. The rest of their blood sugar problems or other bodily problems will be nutritional.

If someone does not have a galbladder, they need to supplement with digestive enzymes and bile to replace this function. It does not require a licensed practitioner to prescribe or sell digestive enzymes. We do not call this "missing galbladder disease." In type 1 a function is missing. A treatment will not bring it back, and so it will not be cured. We can replace the function without ever referencing a disease.

Bone & joint, and the long list of related calcium deficiency problems, do not require medicine. Or surgery. Birth defects do not require medicine. For that matter, birth really shouldn't either.

The only things we have encountered so far that deserve the legal title of disease, are infections.

6. Digestion Diseases.

Healthy digestion is required for a healthy body. Correcting digestion alone can turn the average person's wellbeing around. If there is a digestive problem, the ability for the body to absorb nutrients will be compromised. We have already seen nutrient deficiencies as one of the most important aspects of what we call "disease."

A digestive problem left uncorrected is likely to lead directly to enough symptoms to be called a disease.

Some digestive problems are called diseases themselves. I include these in my list of *Fake Diseases* because it makes absolutely no sense to call a digestive problem a disease. If you add sand to the gasoline before you put it in your car, the car will have a problem. Its performance will be impacted immediately, measurably, and noticeably. It will make zero sense to call this a disease.

If you cleaned out the pipes and put clean gasoline in, the car will run fine. But you would sound foolish to claim that you have cured your car of a disease.

And it would be criminal for a mechanic monopoly to charge you an arm and a leg to fix it. It would be much worse if that profession couldn't even fix it. They just kept it for testing indefinitely, removing more and more parts until it couldn't possibly drive. But insurance still paid.

Imagine if mechanics operated like doctors.

Here are some of the digestive problems and diseases, all of which are mechanical:

- acid reflux
- athlete's foot
- celiac disease
- Chron's disease
- constipation
- dermatitis
- diarrhea
- diverticulitis
- food sensitivities
- gas
- heart burn
- hiatal hernia
- indigestion
- irritable bowel
- leaky gut
- jock itch
- allergies/seasonal allergies
- thrush
- ulcerative colitis
- yeast infections

The yeast infections and other fungal problems show up here because the digestive environment is the foundation of the immune environment. A digestive problem will most likely lead to an immune problem, and a proclivity to various infections like ear, sinus, respiratory, or urinary tract, as well as fungus, which appears in the symptoms of itches and smells, and bumps or dents under the skin or nails.

The fungus, bacteria, virus, and parasites of all kinds, are always there, it seems. No matter where we are on Earth, if we have an unhealthy internal environment, we are likely to develop some kind of infection. This point becomes more important as we move through all of the physical diseases and into the more scary pandemics.

The first major nutrient absorption that will be impacted by a digestive problem are the "good fats." In our camp, all fats are good unless they are burned or oxidized. Oxidized fat or oil is called "rancid" in the books.

Since a digestive problem can lead directly to tissue damage, inflammation, and pain, we get most of the list above as a direct consequence. But we don't catch these things. These are not diseases. These are plumbing issues, not doctor issues. It is not a medicinal problem, or even a nutritional deficiency problem. The problems above are caused by eating the wrong foods.

But more sinister are the resulting deficiency problems and so-called diseases. Since the fat category is the first most likely deficiency to appear in the form of symptoms throughout the body, we should be familiar with the following list:

- acne
- alopecia
- Alzheimer's disease
- asthma
- blood clots
- brittle hair
- cardiovascular disease
- cracked heals
- dementia
- eczema
- fibromyalgia
- gallstones
- growth retardation
- infertility
- kidney dysfunction
- low libido
- low sperm count
- miscarriage
- multiple sclerosis, amyotrophic lateral sclerosis, Huntington's disease, Parkinson's disease
- muscular dystrophy[viii]
- PMS
- psoriasis

The blood sugar, digestion, and "good fat problem" lists combined are the majority of health complaints that people come to us about. And they are usually connected. Most people with one category of problem will have something in another category. Many of them are very serious, life ruining or life ending. Even just one can ruin your life effectively. Constant stomach pain is miserable. It is impossible to enjoy life in such pain.

Many of the things on these lists are uncomfortable, inconvenient, and embarrassing. Of course people want to get rid of these problems. But when they are labeled a disease, or we go to an allopathic practitioner with one of these problems, the treatment offered will usually make the problem worse. Unless they give "alternative" advice, which is unlikely.

The allopathic toolkit for dealing with digestive problems consists of:

- stomach acid lowering tablets
- stomach acid lowering pharmaceutical drugs
- removing parts of the intestines
- choking the stomach with a band, inserted surgically
- removing the stomach
- removing the problematic kidney/gal bladder/liver/appendix
- that's pretty much it.

This sounds too simple to be real. Do doctors really think like this? Well, not really. They have multiple barriers to understanding digestive problems because of the way they are taught about the body – the allopathic way. I genuinely think they just can't see any other way to deal with these problems. This is literally all they know.

Our view is that the body requires all of its organs. Removing any of them will be a problem and shorten lifespan. It also doesn't address the original problem.

The body also requires healthy stomach acid. In our experience, if a person is on stomach acid lowering drugs (proton pump inhibitors, or PPIs), they have very little chance of any improvement. There is not much we can do for them. They can't absorb our products or digest food correctly without a strong stomach acid.

Getting off PPIs can be miserable. It can take weeks. People are often tempted just to take the pill after a few days because of the stomach pain, but if they keep taking the pill they will continue not producing stomach acid. Health will be harder and harder to attain.

Advice on easing this process is in the notes at the back of the book.[ix]

As alternative practitioners, we cannot tell people whether or not they should take drugs. The easiest thing for me to say is, "I wouldn't." I wouldn't take a drug that prevents my stomach from working properly.

We can also tell people that they can take whatever advice they like. They don't have to take their doctor's advice. Some drugs have withdrawal effects. This information is readily available online. The advice usually given is that those drugs with withdrawal concerns should be weaned.

Any other drug type we can basically get around. All drugs cause side effects, but we can still feed the body the right stuff it needs to heal itself, as long as it can be absorbed. PPIs just interfere with the whole process. It's impossible to digest correctly on them. I hope that's clear.

One of my many health problems growing up was chronic stomach pain. I would never have known that the food I was eating was the only reason I was in stomach pain. I wouldn't have known because my doctor didn't tell me. He said to take stomach acid lowering tablets called *Tums*. The next option was proton pump inhibitor drugs, which stop the stomach from working properly.

Allopathic professionals are taught that when there is a problem in the body, the way to "manage" this is to block, stop, remove, or kill something in the body. They don't have the language, the education, or the technology to "support" the body. Everything in their toolkit regarding digestion aims to stop a process in the body. It is appropriate for syphilis, but not stomach pain.

This point is excessively important.

For a profession that only knows how to block things, you would think they would see the obvious solution to a digestive problem. In most cases, they need to block the wrong foods from going down the hatch. That's it.

Most other cases, they need more salt. Salt is required to make stomach acid. Stomach acid is required to break down food in the stomach, before it goes into the intestines to be absorbed.

Doctors messed up big time by erroneously blocking humans from consuming salt. Much of the stomach pain on Earth is a direct result of this. In the health business we make no money by promoting salt, but the products we are trying to sell our customers also need to be absorbed through the same route as food. If they have a digestive problem, not only will they have a health issue, but we will have a problem trying to help them. They need to absorb the nutrients.

We love to point out that there isn't a farmer on Earth who could be profitable without providing their animals with unlimited salt. As much as they want. Any less and they will have a problem. The body is smarter than we are. A pig body is smarter than a human doctor. It knows exactly how much salt it wants. When it has had enough, it will stop licking. The horse or cow or goat cannot physically lick "too much." You could hold their head down in front of the salt block, and it will not lick it.

It is the same way in humans. As polite as you try to be, you will not be able to consume a meal that is "too salty." It will be one of the most repulsive things you've ever experienced. If you force this into your mouth, you will likely vomit.

It would be rude of me just to point out that digestion problems are not actually diseases, without stating how to correct a digestive problem, and the first place to start is the salt. We have an extremely sensitive meter for salt. Things can become "too salty" with just a few extra shakes of the salt shaker, but it is delicious until that point. The moment we have enough, it becomes repulsive.

We teach people to act like livestock. Our salt meter is likely out of balance with our conscious brain. We often mistake a salt craving for a potato chip or candy bar craving. We mistake the body asking for salt and water for "food and drink."

I'm not recommending a salt lick in the kid's bedroom. I recommend what we call "the salt flush", which is a glass of water with 3 heaping tablespoons of salt in it. Mix it well. Natural salts are best for this but it would work with table salt.

It should be cloudy. Take one tiny sip. It should be the saltiest thing you've ever tasted. But chances are, it is stimulating, refreshing, and tastes surprisingly good.

With each small sip you get more and more used to it. If we are low on salt, it might be the best thing we've ever tasted.

Most people can only take a few sips, and that means they're not low on salt. It still feels nice, but it is very quickly too salty. If someone can drink a lot of the glass, or the whole thing, they are very low on salt.

If someone has had a digestive problem, they will probably be able to drink a fair bit, or the whole glass. If someone is experiencing stomach pain, as they drink more of the salty water they should feel soothing relief in the stomach.

They may be driven to the bathroom for a vigorous expulsion. This potential is where we got the name "salt *flush*" from.

There is a potential for temporary discomfort after a salt flush. If the person could only drink a bit of it, then there should be no negative effect. But if they could drink a lot, or the whole glass, they could experience diarrhea, a migraine, a flu-like 24-48 hour experience, or they could vomit. Each is temporary, but the body will continue to adjust for weeks if the person has been severely limiting salt.

Unfortunately, if the body needed a lot of salt, and it experienced a reaction like above, our recommendation is to try the flush again a couple of days later. Fill up another glass and see how much you can drink. It should be much less than the first time. If there is an uncomfortable side effect, it should be much less than the first time.

Repeat every 2-3 days until you can only take a few sips. That is where we should be at any given time – topped up.

Now you should be in tune with your salt meter. Henceforth, you should be able to give your body exactly how much salt it needs. We wake up dehydrated, and some salty water in the morning is one of the best things we can do to re-hydrate. Most of us will find that just a few shakes of a salt shaker is what our body is looking for. Many of us feel that water without a bit of salt in it now tastes stale and boring.

All you have to do in your daily life is use enough salt on your food or added into your water, coffee, or tea, and you will have the raw material needed to make stomach acid.[x] Some foods are harder to digest than others, meat particularly, and more-so the more it is cooked. Use more salt on these foods. Salt the food until you can taste the salt. "Salt to taste" doesn't mean salt as much as you feel like, it means add salt until you can taste the salt and then stop.

Now that the stomach can do its job, we still have to make sure we're not putting the wrong foods in. It's more important to cover the bad foods, because the list is much shorter than the good foods. In our business, we really don't care what you eat, as long as it's not the bad foods.

Grains will be the biggest problem in most people's diet. We would put special emphasis on the "gluten" grains: wheat, barley, and rye. And we would include oats and quinoa on the "definitely avoid" list.[xi]

It tends to take about two weeks of total grain avoidance, like sugar, to break the addictive attachment to these foods. There can be withdrawal experience in the first few weeks avoiding gluten particularly. But it is worth it. If you had anything on the lists in the digestive or blood sugar or good fat deficiency lists, it might disappear in a few weeks or months, just by removing these grains from the diet.

This information actually isn't that great for our business model. We have to, in good conscience, give all of the information we have to offer. We offer supplement advice, which we sell, but we also offer food advice, because food can be causing the problem.

The problem for us is, it is very common for our prospective customers to walk away with the food and salt information, and completely turn around their health. Without buying products from us. This is how important digestion can be.

If someone is in disbelief about gluten or grains, or they believe their doctor who told them there is nothing to worry about, and to just eat the food groups, this is the pitch we offer:

If someone avoids gluten completely for 14 days

1. they will probably feel better by the 14th day
2. if they are in any doubt, we recommend consuming gluten with each meal on the 15th day

The pain endured by re-introducing gluten is usually enough to make the point.

It is not a guarantee that two weeks without gluten will completely convince a non-believer, but it is very likely. A whole month, or three, is a much more reasonable trial.

There could be other problematic compounds in the food, but it is most likely that these grains are the cause of the constipation, diarrhea, migraines, leaky gut, irritable bowel, and possibly even the eczema, psoriasis and other soft tissue problems.

Heart burn should go away with a salt flush, but it will come back by eating harmful foods like grains. If the stomach can break down food, with a strong stomach acid, chronic stomach pain should not occur.[xii] Acute stomach pain is likely with overeating – relieve with a salt flush and decrease portion size in the future. As you improve digestion and health, you will not be able to eat as much as you used to.

Intestines can take a long time to fully heal. But the longer someone avoids problematic foods, particularly gluten and other grains, the better they should feel.

These two things, adding salt and removing gluten, will help anyone who tries, and in most cases they won't need to do anything else in order to experience healthy digestion.

My favorite thing to add on top of this, in the short term, is diatomaceous earth (DE). Diatomaceous earth is ground shell flour. It is one of the cheapest and most effective health products available on Earth.

I first learned of it in chickens. Our hens were not producing enough eggs. We were advised to add either diatomaceous earth or oyster shells, as both contain nutrients required for egg production. Full production resumed within days.

I learned that it is also commonly used in dogs and cats, to kill worms and other parasites in the body. No drugs needed. Diatomaceous earth kills bugs and bad bacteria inside the body and outside. I plug up ant holes with it and they never return.

Some health practitioners, alternative and mainstream, claim that using diatomaceous earth (or psyllium husk, or bentonite clay), can damage the intestines or cause malabsorption of nutrients. In our experience with hair analysis, we have been unable to find any evidence of this. We have countless positive testimonials and no uncomfortable side effects that I am aware of other than a strong bowel movement. The worst case scenario is that the DE doesn't work.

In addition to attracting pathogens and neutralizing them, diatomaceous earth "clears out the pipes" as it moves through the guts. We often deal with very overweight people. Some of them have reported losing 20lbs through their bowels because of diatomaceous earth. This is in one day. Many of us are carrying a lot of weight in the intestines that wants to come out. I assume at least that our body would want it out.

When correcting digestion, I highly recommend adding two heaping tablespoons of diatomaceous earth to that morning salty glass of water. Don't use any metal. Use a plastic, wood, ceramic, or glass cup and stir stick. Metal is said to neutralize the electrical charge which is said to be the active component of the stuff. Apparently stainless steel is fine, but don't chance it. If the electric charge is neutralized, it basically becomes just sand, and will not give the desired results. If the product isn't working at all, the manufacturer probably used metal. Diatomaceous earth has a very noticeable effect, and you will feel quickly whether it is working or not.

For best results do this 2 or 3 times a day for 1-3 months.

Also, don't breathe the dust. It's never good to breathe dust.

There are two other things worth mentioning here for correcting digestion. Doing all of these at once practically guarantees a quick route to healthy digestion.

The first is probiotics. These do not need to be supplemented, but it can definitely help to add them at the beginning. Some strains can produce a negative reaction. If this happens, switch to a product with different strains. Many brands are marketed to have less problematic strains in them.

Seeking to eat fermented foods containing probiotics is a good idea. These foods are easy to digest, and so they are already a good idea for someone dealing with a digestive problem. And by providing more good bacteria, this is providing more of the raw material we need to correctly digest, absorb, and expel food. These foods can be eaten daily.

The last thing I want to mention about digestion is digestive enzymes. Here it is necessary to point out that, if someone has had their gallbladder removed, that person needs to supplement with digestive enzymes for the rest of their lives.

When food is broken down in the stomach and driven into the intestines, it is met with several digestive enzymes which are responsible for certain proteins. The gallbladder is a little sack that releases bile containing some of these critical enzymes. Without these enzymes, several critical nutrients, including the good fats, cannot be absorbed.

We saw the horrible list of fat deficiency problems at the start of the chapter. All of these can be caused by a lack of enzymes. A good enzyme product will contain a spread of enzymes, as well as bile (ox bile usually). It should also contain some Cl compound, likely betaine HCl. Stomach acid is mainly HCl. Like salt, betaine HCl serves to provide the raw material for the acid in stomach acid.

Someone without a gallbladder must do this, or it is impossible to correctly digest any food containing fat. But the rest of us can also benefit by using digestive enzymes short term. Taking one or two in the morning with that salty water is a great way to further encourage healthy digestion.

Taking 1-2 more enzyme capsules a few minutes before meals will further improve the odds that the meal will be digested uneventfully.

If you have a gallbladder, this should only be short term. We produce our own enzymes in our body. When we are digesting correctly, properly nourished, and not overburdening our body with too much food, we will produce sufficient enzymes.

There are other things that can help digestion and soothe stomachs. But these 5 things (using salt, staying away from problematic grains, using diatomaceous earth, probiotics, and digestive enzymes) are a very powerful combination. Doing any one of them will likely show improvement. The more, the better.[xiii]

Up until this point most of the discussion has been largely mechanical. From here on in, we are going to cover more complicated subjects like cancer and autoimmune diseases. But we have laid all the necessary groundwork.

The reason these next subjects are more complicated, is because there is more than one contributing factor. One of those factors is likely to be digestion. As we know, a digestive problem is likely to lead to a blood sugar problem, and so this is also likely to show up in a person with cancer or an autoimmune problem.

The non-infectious diseases we have covered so far, as we have seen, can be explained directly. Something is missing or it is in the way. Well, we also don't catch cancer or an autoimmune disease, and though they are more complicated than a bone problem or a birth defect, they share the same roots. They are the more serious consequence of a body that isn't working properly – a body that isn't healthy, a lack of ease.

What does a body need to be healthy? Enough of the essential nutrients to do the many jobs properly, and a clean environment to do it in. This is how the wrong foods, or nutrient deficiencies, have caused every non-infectious problem we have encountered so far.

7. Cancer.

Cancer is definitely dis-ease, a lack of health. But to be a disease is to be classified as something requiring treatment from a licensed medical practitioner.

We don't catch cancer, and as far as the mainstream medical world is concerned, we do not cure cancer either. If a cancer patient, by any route, ends up losing their symptoms, or improve on whichever measurements they are using, they can only be deemed "in remission."

There currently is not the legal terminology or framework to deem any cancer as curable. Doctors don't speak like that. They are not supposed to. And neither are we.

If we were all in agreement that the word disease means a lack of ease, then this would be no problem. But we are taught about diseases in reference to almost any health problem, and we are all operating under a system which empowers only one profession to deal with them all.

We could just call infections "infections", and change the legal status of "treatment of disease" to mean "treatment of infection." That could be left in the jurisdiction of the allopathic medical profession. This ensures the appropriate prescription of pharmaceutical medication required to treat such problems. We could call all the other health problems something else.

There would not be a need for this book in that case. We would treat infections as diseases, by seeking medical intervention, and we would treat everything else as a multi factored nutritional consequence. We could call them diseases and treat them by correcting our food and nutrition. We could call them something else if we choose. Or we could use the already existing framework in animal nutrition to correct our eating and nutrient intake, and forget the names of these health problems.

The animal breeder who supplements correctly will never have to deal with any strange named diseases, or cancer. Benign growths, or "tumors", are common in older animals, but they do not die from these growths, and there is no sense in calling them a tumor, because tumors are more widely understood as a form of cancer.

Cancer is not one thing. I don't believe cancer is even *a* thing, to be honest. Cancer seems to be the name they give when the body is failing rapidly and catastrophically, and doctors can't figure it out. In my view, cancer cannot exist unless multiple things are going wrong in the body. Since it is not caused by one thing, and since it can show up in any system in the body, this is why I do not think it is useful to view it as *a* thing.

It is also not reversed by any one thing, but we will get more into that later.

The language is important to start with. Syphilis is *a thing*. It's a bug. It's a noun. By our description of diabetes, diabetes is not a noun, it is a verb. A verb is an action or a process. Arthritis is not a thing, it's what happens when things are missing. It would be more appropriate to speak of a person who is diabetes-*ing* or arthritis-*ing,* because that would describe the dis-ease as a process.

When a human goes to a doctor, and is given a Latin name for their list of symptoms, they are liable to walk away believing they *have* a disease. Have is a possessive word. A noun is a thing that can be possessed. But most of this book is not about nouns. A virus is a noun, but cancer is a poorly defined verb.

If one thinks they *have* a disease, they might speak of themselves in this way: "I *am* a diabetic." Claiming this identity cannot be helpful for the solution, because the noun disease entitles this person to the care only of the allopathic professions. Since they view all disease in this noun form, they only treat "things." Worse, they tend to treat "things" with other "things" that are invariably harmful, such as drugs and surgeries and radiation. Since diabetes and cancer and osteoporosis and acne are not nouns, this treatment is useless, expensive, and potentially dangerous or deadly.

On a psychological level, it is not helpful to believe you are diseased. I was born with birth defects and pain. I don't think of it as a disease. I didn't catch it from my mother. She was missing some things during pregnancy. That's it.

Worse, since the "cure" word is practically unattainable to a patient with chronic disease, the person might be tempted to identify as a disease patient or survivor for the rest of their lives. Why not believe we can turn our health around by our own choices? Why not believe we can heal?

This is a great time to focus on "belief" for a moment. Behind every therapy there is a belief that it will work, or a belief that it will not work. Your mind is likely more powerful than the therapy. If you believe it will work, or help, it will probably help, at least temporarily. If you do not believe it will work, it will probably seem like a waste of time.

When it comes to people who claim to no longer have cancer, a lot of these testimonies are found inside content that is focusing on belief. A lot of this is religious. People believe they have the power to heal. They refuse the mainstream therapy, or they believe so strongly that the therapy will work because God has endowed their doctors, that they survive normal healthy longevity.

Atheists will call this placebo. Whatever we call it, I believe that belief is one of the most important components to both health and longevity. I say this from research into the placebo effect, spiritual healings, and also from experience with real people and chronic disease. Super old people in interviews really don't seem worried about much. They believe it's going to be okay. They've seen it all before. They've outlived 6 husbands. They don't believe what the doctors today say because they've seen the mainstream opinion change many times throughout their lifetimes. In their youth, doctors might still have believed "bad humors" were the root cause of all disease. They don't have to have a happy-go-lucky attitude, they basically just have to believe that they will wake up tomorrow.

The oldest people we can find on Earth tend not to have ever seen a "real" doctor. The point here is that it seems crucial to believe that life will go on, to believe that we will get over the sickness, heal the wound, or provide our body with the material it needs to have a decently functioning body.

They say having a pet at home makes it more likely that you will make it out of hospital. The active ingredient here seems to be *desire*. People who *want* to get better are likely to.

If belief is essential to good health, happiness, and longevity, then surely the belief that "I am *diseased*", must be destructive. If you believe the only hope you have is with an allopathic pharmacologist or surgeon, then your thoughts must be quite bleak. Might as well write the will, right?

As we cover every successful aspect of healing I have encountered, it should be assumed that belief is a required ingredient. Belief and desire together will accomplish most things in life. In animals, this does not really matter. You give them what they need and they're fine. I don't think livestock have a negative attitude about treatments or the belief that they're not going to make it because they "have" a disease.

I have never seen a cancer patient who had only one category of problem. Since we have mentioned belief, it is also worth mentioning that diseases of attitude often coincide with physical ailments. I have also never met a cancer survivor with a bad attitude. If anything, their experience has enhanced their self awareness, gratitude, and positive philosophies.

This means that people in pain, or people identifying with a disease, often have a bad attitude as well. This really boils down to belief systems. Cynical, pessimistic, and nihilistic beliefs will pollute life in many ways, including I think in the chances that one will thrive physically or not. I have heard of many people with such a strong positive attitude that they essentially believed their way out of chronic pain or illness. Faith *can* heal.

Think about it. Someone with a "what's the point?" attitude is un-likely to even take a proper therapy regiment seriously. Lifestyle changes require discipline to implement. Good nutrition requires money and attention. The cynic is too busy being cynical to be healthy. "I guess I'll just go in for the chemo... sigh."

Allopathic treatment is offered in a way that doesn't ask much from the patient other than obedience. Just show up, get in the machine, lay down on this, cough twice, take these pills and call me in two weeks. The lazy person is a perfect victim for this sales pitch. Our alternative pitch asks for quite a bit of commitment, and the cus-tomer has to pay for it, not insurance. But it might actually help. Most of the cynics will likely never know – but they might get their knees replaced. At least insurance pays.

The Buddhists talk about the curse of the 2 arrows, or the 2 thorns. The pain is the first arrow. Stressing about the pain is the second.

A guy gets the flu, that's one arrow. But he's really stressed about missing work. There's an important project on a tight deadline. His absence will surely cause a delay in the production schedule. His many bosses are not going to like this.

The second arrow can be avoided. We are all going to catch a few thorns in life. Winters will come and some years will be worse than others. Bugs will get us now and then. People we know and love will die. If we slack on our health, pains and symptoms will appear. But if we believe we are helpless against this, we will experience second and third arrows, and maybe more. If we identify as a vic-tim of a disease we will, for certain, experience many more arrows for the duration of our anguish.

There is a lot of stress involved in being diagnosed with and treated for a disease. The seriousness of the diagnosis itself, the waiting, the testing, the conversations around the dinner table. The initial therapies and side effects. Maybe some improvement, maybe not. Doctors who aren't all that confident about any of this. Doctors who, if you ask them with a straight face: "what are my chances?" if they are honest they will answer: "not good."

None of this provides faith. None of this encourages healing. All of this is stressful. Stress is the opposite of relaxation. Relaxation is required for healing. The uncertainty and grimness surrounding "disease" provide nothing but fear and stress – the opposite of faith and rest – and this is anathema to healing. All of this is reinforced by media dramas that portray "fighting" cancer with poisons and machines, and we all know that even if we survive we are likely to be greatly damaged by the treatment. (People don't lose their hair and vomit daily because of cancer, those are side effects of cancer *treatment*).

An honest and informed doctor knows that the chances of surviving chemotherapy or radiation are very slim. Any confidence they exhume is probably either from ignorance, or it is simply an act. As an alternative practitioner, I know that if someone has already done chemo or radiation, their chances are still not very good, even if they change their eating and supplementation immediately. They have already been excessively damaged by mainstream treatments, and I don't downplay the seriousness of their situation. If someone came to us *before* a mainstream treatment, I will have a lot of confidence that they can fully reverse their problem, but if they come to us after, our advice is now to take several *extra* products and take the food advice very seriously, if they are to have any hope of reversal.

We try to remedy all of the damage they have experienced with understanding and confidence, but we are in a rough position with people from the start.

One of the most unfortunate aspects of being in the alternative health business is that most of our customers only find us after they have been wandering around the marketplace looking for answers already. Since the monopoly in the medical marketplace is held by the allopathic professions, most of our prospective customers have already undergone some form of mainstream treatment.

So they already had a problem, then they took it to someone who made the problem worse, and now we not only have to help them, but also teach them to think about the entire process of disease differently than they've ever heard. It's not an easy business.

In the case of cancer, that "treatment," as usual, is mostly just pharmaceutical drugs that attack the body in some way. We all know the consequences of this innocently named "chemo*therapy.*" In my view, this is the most damaging part about cancer. It's not the cancer, it's the fact that the human has had to endure such chemical punishment. Second arrow via doctor.

On my end, I know the person with a diagnosis of cancer needs a lot more support than the average person. Recommended nutritional doses are designed for *healthy* people, and sick people need much more. They need a longer to-do list than the average person, and we would encourage them to take it much more seriously.

I rarely encounter anyone who has done radiation "therapy" these days. Usually it's just chemo. They tell me it has become quite widely believed that radiation is much more harmful than helpful. I would agree and am grateful that it is apparently becoming a rare choice of treatment. Of course this is being phased out quietly by the allopathic world who promoted radiation as one of the only possible options for a cancer patient to survive.

Notice I haven't really differentiated between cancers. To me, it doesn't matter whether it's breast cancer or blood cancer. Blood is much more serious of course. But they are caused by the same combination of problems, in my estimation. We alternative people don't have "chemo" things to use, or fancy machines, so it really doesn't matter what terminology we use, as long as we stay away from the forbidden "treatment", or "cure."

This is fine. We don't need to "treat" cancer, because cancer isn't a thing. Syphilis needs to be treated. If cancer is the result of a very unhealthy body, then we can encourage a healthy body in a number of ways.

We have already explored digestion improvement. This, combined with good food habits and nutrient supplementation can encourage healthy blood sugar. A consequence of a blood sugar problem is a circulation problem, and so a consequence of healthy blood sugar is likely to be healthy circulation as well.

Healthy circulation is required for the correct delivery of nutrients, oxygen and sugar to each cell, and to transport the waste effectively out of the system. A circulation problem is a big problem.

I believe every cancer has something to do with circulation. Digestion could be at the start of this chain of events. Nutrient deficiency is likely at the start, and guaranteed once a problem has arisen. Some legal claims have been won regarding specific nutrients and cancer benefits.[xiv] These, in our view, are simply essential nutrients and antioxidants that are doing their job. Their job is to keep the body healthy. A healthy body does not have cancer. One of the potential consequences of an unhealthy body, is cancer.

You can see the hoops we have to run through even to explain cancer in a way that begins to make sense. Calling it a disease never made sense if we are supposed to think about diseases as a thing requiring treatment.

On top of avoiding foods like gluten that screw up the digestive system, it is wise to avoid foods that are known to increase the likelihood of developing cancer. The words here are again important. A lot of people are these days talking about meat *causing cancer*. But technically we can only demonstrate certain foods as increasing the likelihood that a person will develop some kind of cancer. Some meats are on our bad list, and we will cover them.

Top of our bad list, after grains, is liquid oils. Oil is present in every tissue in nature. It is protected from oxidation by the skin, peel, or shell. Once the protective barrier is broken or the plant or animal dies, the oil begins to "oxidize." Oxidized oil is called "rancid." The name sounds gross because it is. It is rotten fat. Oxidized fats contain a large amount of "free-radical" oxygen particles. Unstable oxygen particles.[xv]

The body uses an array of compounds called "anti-oxidants" to combat free-radical particles. Some of these are also considered essential nutrients, such as zinc or vitamin C. Some antioxidants, such as glutathione, we produce ourselves in almost every cell in the body. This master antioxidant requires one of the more important minerals, selenium, to function.

This is mainstream textbook stuff, but it isn't applied generally in the human population or in allopathic medical recommendations. This is because this is not medicine. Selenium is a nutrient, not a medicine. Allopathic professionals are not required to learn anything about nutrition.

Nutrients are not able to be patented. So the development end of this industry does not have much to gain by pursuing selenium "treatment." The only possible outcome in giving more of this essential nutrient is healthier patients, which is not very profitable for an industry that legally only "treats" disease.

Interesting that doctors are not supposed to sell products. And they are not supposed to be paid to recommend drugs either. They are supposed to be unbiased professionals. But if they recommended simple nutritional strategies such as food avoidances and nutrient supplementation, in almost every type of disease they would never need to see their patients again.

We definitely would not need as many doctors on standby to try to deal with the everyday ailments that affect the average person. People wouldn't be getting joint replacement surgeries if they were rebuilding their skeletons with nutrition. People wouldn't be getting stomach and intestinal surgeries because they would stop eating the foods causing the stomach and intestinal problems. People wouldn't be getting cancer treatments with drugs and radiation because they would be supporting a healthy body, and a healthy body doesn't have cancer.

This point is already obvious to much of my audience. If the job of a doctor was to help people get healthy, they would put most of the profession out of work. I'm allowed to sell products. In exchange for not being allowed to "treat" people, I am given free license to help people get healthy.

If my customers fail to get results, they will not buy my products again. Since I expect most of my income to come from residual customers – people who buy the same products over and over, tell their friends and so on – it is in my financial interests to help them any way I can.

If my customers achieve perfect health, I will make the most money from them, and in my experience healthy people buy more products than sick people! It is interesting to compare this to the allopathic professions, depending for their business on steady and growing sickness. As businesses operate on inflationary assumptions, the medical profession within the capitalist system must also expect "growth."

This means more sick people. Without more sick people, the medical industry will be at a loss. This is basic but important, especially when we are talking about huge industries like cancer, diabetes, and bone/joint diseases.

Free-radicals are produced in the body when we exercise, breathe, and when we digest things. When we use energy, basically. It is a natural byproduct of life. In the normal amount of exercise and digestion, and the adequate nutrient and antioxidant levels available, the body is able to deal with the regular burden of free-radical damage.

In addition, with all the nutrients present and a good digestive environment, all the cells in the body are able to regenerate with only a small margin of error. This accounts for gradual aging, but it does not account for disease, unless there is much more than a normal amount of degeneration.

So, free-radicals can damage cells. That's natural. We regenerate and move on. Too many free-radicals can quickly be a big problem, especially in a modern environment critically lacking many of the essential nutrients, and antioxidants.

Recently, health foods have begun marketing products without oil. This is good, though it is still hard to avoid oil if eating any packaged or processed foods.

There are other sources of free-radicals. Car exhaust, industrial activity, and other established pollutants all result in a free-radical burden on the body.

Air quality in major cities has been improving in recent years. But it is not air that poses the most serious threat. We can't breathe as much as we can eat. A small serving of oxidized oil is much more harmful than the particles in the air. Fried food is much more dangerous than smoking in this equivocation.

Baked potato skins are also on our list, for this same reason, an end result of "too much damage to compensate." If you eat baked potato skins regularly you will have a problem. Boiled is fine. Raw is probably not fine but I don't recommend trying it either way.

One baked potato skin, nice and crispy, has a large ratio of free-radicals per gram of total weight. One baked potato skin weighs much, much more than an entire carton of cigarettes when smoked. Smoke is bad for the number of chemicals in it which ultimately lead to this same consequence: the need for much more nutrition and antioxidants to attempt to deal with the free-radical damage. But smoke doesn't weigh much. So even if it was 100% free-radicals, it would still be hard to compare to a food source.

Since there is much more weight of these toxic particles in food than in smoke, eating is our primary source of free-radicals.

This is why many people with lung cancer do not smoke, and never did smoke. It is also why primitive people could live with an *open fire pit inside their homes*, and not get lung cancer. Cancer in general, and lung cancer in particular, is a rather new phenomenon. Surely we didn't have the diagnostic capacity a hundred or more years ago that we now have, but very generally cancer was not a recognized problem until the 20th century. The mainstream medical world has no idea what causes, prevents, or reverses cancer or heart disease or diabetes (the top three causes of death in America), and so they have looked for explanations all over the place. They latched onto smoking, and "second-hand" smoking, as well as dietary fat and lack of exercise, to try to explain the increasing prevalence of these diseases.[xvi] By and large, the public has listened to their advice, and both smoking and dietary fat intakes have decreased dramatically over several decades – yet cancer, heart disease, diabetes, and so on have not declined significantly at all.

The major sources of these same types of chemicals in cigarettes are in foods and how we cook them. Standing over a deep fryer or a stove top pan cooking something with oil, will likely lead to more free-radicals in your lungs in minutes than you would get from weeks or months of heavy smoking. This is weight. Oil particles are heavy. Potato skins add up. And the next ones on our list are heavy sources too.

When we start talking about the weight of a bowl of deep fried onion rings, in my estimation it is physically impossible to smoke that much. The person would die of smoke inhalation, not cancer. You can't smoke anywhere near as much as you can eat.

Well-done red meat, or any burned animal fat, or any charred food, is also a major source of free-radicals. We cannot consume enough nutrients, or antioxidants, to combat the damage of regular consumption of these foods. We recommend you keep your steaks to a maximum of medium-rare. It is okay to stew or bake red meats to well-done, but only if the temperature is low. Boiling water doesn't go beyond 100°C, and as a general rule "low and slow" (low temp, long time), is best for cooking meats to avoid burning the fats or producing too many problematic compounds. Medium-rare steaks will still have some of these compounds, but they are kept to a reasonable level – any more than medium-rare is just too much for the body to deal with.

Processed meats containing nitrogen compounds are on our list as well, for the same end result: free-radical damage. This is most of our list actually.[xvii] These major sources of damage to the body bring us to the heart of what I believe cancer to be.

Free-radicals demand resources in the form of antioxidants for the body to attempt to deal with. This process also requires essential nutrients as the spark plugs involved in these antioxidant functions.

As the demand for antioxidants increases, as does the demand for the essential nutrients involved. These nutrients are also required for numerous other functions in the body, including a healthy immune system and cell regeneration.

If the body has to make choices about how to devote limited resources, it is likely to attempt to deal with the most pressing situation at hand.

If the most serious ongoing situation in the body is a constant attack by the over consumption of free-radicals and other toxic compounds, then the body is forced to divert significant resources just to deal with the daily damage from the diet.

This leaves those other important functions hanging. What is the immune system to do if there is not even enough nutrients available to handle breakfast?

Since essential nutrients are required for every function in the body, this type of situation can lead to a problem anywhere in the body. I believe it is this state, this nutrient deprived free-radical war zone, that results in problems that are called either cancer, or an autoimmune disease. We will cover autoimmune problems next, but I wanted to mention that I don't think there is much difference, other than the fact that cancer is localized and an immune problem is generalized. Cancer occurs in one place (and it can spread), and immune problems are not located in any one part of the body. Both are end results of an overall unhealthy body.

Many people say "sugar feeds cancer." I think this idea makes more sense in view of this explanation. Sugar also demands significant nutrients, produces free-radicals, and blood sugar problems lead to numerous other problems. In my experience, nearly every cancer patient I have dealt with had some obvious blood sugar symptom on their list of problems. Whether they had that before their cancer diagnosis and treatment, I can't be sure – I usually only see them after.

Having said all of this, now the experiences I will share next will hopefully make more sense.

In my time in the business, I have met many people who told me they had cancer, and that they no longer do. I have heard a huge number of things attributed to this success. I have noticed some commonalities.

The most common story I have heard, emphasizes fasting. This means, not eating.

All food requires nutrients and energy to digest. There are toxic byproducts to digestion that the body must also devote nutrients and energy to dispose of. Even good food costs the body to digest it. Too much food is one of the most common problems in the modern world, in my opinion.

Not eating immediately lifts this burden – and you can't eat any of the bad foods if you are not eating at all. Nutrients that might have been used to digest, can be used to maintain and repair the body, or support the immune system.

I didn't mention fasting in the digestion section because I wanted to mention it here. Fasting for short periods (intermittent fasting), or longer periods, is one of the easiest ways to aid digestion. If there is a digestion problem, it is highly likely that the conveyor belt of our digestive system is overloaded with food.

Even 24/hr diners close at least once a year to clean out the kitchen. Fasting allows the body to deal with material that needs to get out. Fasting can make people feel wonderful and light. Bowel movements can continue for days without food, proving how behind schedule the system has been.

Fasting can also reduce hunger. It is common to find one of the immediate consequences to disciplined fasting is a general decrease in the desire for food. People having trouble controlling portions will find this one of the most useful ways to change this habit.

Fasting can be difficult if a blood sugar problem is present. If you become dizzy or light headed, it is okay to break the fast. Some dried fruit, especially dates, are a quick way to bring up the blood sugar. Eating fat or protein will provide more satisfaction than carbs or sugar, but will not raise the blood sugar as quickly.

Salty water, salty broth, or fruit or vegetable juices will also likely allow a person to dramatically decrease the amount of food burdening their system. Very often we confuse thirst for hunger. As a person improves their overall health and digestion, fasting will become easier and more physically enjoyable. Working on an empty stomach is quite healthy.

Of course we have all heard stories of people who jumped into consuming a majority of their food in juice form, and experienced impressive health improvements. Many of them show no signs of their past diseases, including cancer. We can see why this is one of the things that could contribute to a healthy body.

Juices are concentrated foods. They are easier to digest, and so they require less overall work and more payoff because they are more nutritionally concentrated than solid food.

Since they are more nutritionally dense, they are more satisfying. In this process, we consume less calories. Excess calories burden the system, producing free-radicals when digested.

Juices also tend to not contain the bad foods we've listed so far. Juices should not have gluten, oil, baked potato skins, well-done red meat, burned animal fat, charred food, or processed meats in them. Not the kind of juice I'd like to drink anyway.

To me, this is the main reason why both fasting and juicing show great results in pushing people toward health: They are not the bad foods!

Avoiding the foods that contribute the most damage to the body is probably important if we want to avoid chronic disease. So when a strategy happens to limit the consumption of these foods, there will likely be a lot of success stories.

This also explains why many diets are successful in the short term turnaround of people from catastrophic disease states like cancer. The raw vegans won't be eating any of those things above. If you only eat fruit you are avoiding all of the things above. If you sub-scribe to the paleo diet you are avoiding all of these foods, or most. Any diet that avoids gluten, oil, burned foods, or processed foods, or any combination, will have followers who claim to be in remis-sion from cancer.

And I believe them.

None of this is a "cure", to be clear. These are only some of the things that contribute to stress within the body, and some of the things that ease that stress. Under the belief that the body can maintain and repair itself, this is our main task if we want to active-ly encourage a healthy body.

If there were one magic compound that disappeared the symptoms of cancer, we could call it a cure. The people running for a cure seem to be hoping for something like this. But this will never hap-pen. Since no cancer is caused by one thing, it will never be re-versed by one thing.

Let's focus on the word "stress" for the moment. Free-radical stress is one form of stress. Digestive distress is another. Nutrient deficiency is a stress on the body. There are many forms of stress, all of which contribute to a state of dis-ease. Consequently, strategies that alleviate stress in one form or another are invariably successful in reducing symptoms of an unhealthy body, including cancer.

This is why I have heard so many stories of people who got a serious diagnosis of some kind, and rather than undergo a chemical or surgical procedure that the allopathic professional assured them would be painful and with slim chance of success, they chose to move back home or go on an extended fishing trip instead.

Their reasons differ. Some people said they wanted to spend their last days doing something they enjoyed, catching up with and cherishing time with loved ones, or crossing off things on their bucket list that they always wanted to do.

Some people didn't have the money for conventional treatment, and were forced to do nothing. Many of these people simply just carried on.

Some people were devastated by the news of a terminal illness. They were determined to beat it and they searched for strategies that could help them get healthy. Most of what I have mentioned so far is common knowledge in the alternative health world. A lot of the camps focus on one part or another of the strategies we've mentioned. But the information is there and many people find it on the internet or find us at health shows, conventions, expos, seminars, and Facebook groups.

Anything that relieves stress on the body or mind will be good for the body. A stressed body is not going to be worried about healing. Fight or flight is one state of being, and rest and restore is the other. We cannot be in both modes at the same time.

This is not scientific, it is grandma's recipe. We cannot digest adequately if we are exercising vigorously. We're not supposed to eat before swimming. People stressed about a relationship breakup or a job loss tend to become uninterested in food, or they can eat obsessively. Obsessiveness distracts from feeding the body properly, or distracts from responsibility generally.

By the same token, being given a diagnosis by a medical doctor is often very stressful itself. We are told we have a disease, and then presented some painful options, none of which are promoted with the intention to "cure" the problem.

This fear instilled by the medical profession is in my opinion responsible for quite a lot of unnecessary suffering. One of the positive benefits we should enjoy by seeking professional medical attention, is relief that the responsibility is being handled by someone who knows what they are doing. But if the medical monopoly has mislabeled many things "diseases" just so they can treat them, they might not be able to offer any hope if those problems are not successfully treated by allopathic protocols.

This means, if a drug or surgery can't immediately fix the problem, then the doctor probably can't help. So they can't offer the consolation you would get from somebody who knows what they're doing – since in these cases, they in fact do not know what they are doing.

On top of gaining control over our own digestion and nutrition, it is wise of us to put conscious attention towards rest and relaxation. Here is a short list of things that can encourage relaxation:

- sleep
- hot shower/bath/sauna
- sunbathing
- swimming
- yoga
- hugs/cuddling/massage
- fishing/golfing/other leisure sports or games
- reading
- arts and crafts
- playing with animals
- acupuncture, or any therapy that is relaxing such as sound therapy, aromatherapy, or meditation

Taking all of this into consideration, if I was given a diagnosis of a disease – any disease – I would pick as much of the topics covered so far and implement the strategies. If it was cancer, which is the very serious end of the scale of an unhealthy body, I would do every possible thing on the list that could help "support and promote maintenance and repair" of a healthy body.

If I was determined to live and wasn't messing around, this is exactly what I would do:

I would listen to the advice of the doctor giving me the diagnosis. I would take notes and ask as many questions as possible.

If I was at all considering their advice, I would ask if I could contact a few of their past patients to ask about their experience with the treatment.

Having read up until now I have a good bit of advice to start with. I should remain calm. In fact, after such a stressful and worrisome encounter, I should stop and get in a massage or a sauna or a salt water swim before I go home. Maybe a workout. Maybe a walk by the water.

When I got home, I would hug my wife, tell her I love her, and ask to sit down for a serious conversation.

The tone of this conversation would not be "I've got cancer!"

The tone would be, hunny, my body is clearly overwhelmed and under nourished. We're going to need to get rid of those bad foods we still have in the house. And we're going to need to make sure there is no gluten, oil, or burned food in our diet.

I'm going to stop all the candy and stuff cold turkey until my health is completely on the upswing and my doctor is no longer worried.

I am confident that I can restore my body to health. I will need your help. And I will need to divert a bit more money to health products for at least a few months. This alternative guy I talked to said I should put down at least a few hundred bucks if I want to give it my best shot.

Realistically, if it were me facing losing it all, I'd do more than just the basic essential nutrient recommendation. That's what we're supposed to need to *maintain*. If we're sick, we need more.

I'd first increase the selenium. I wouldn't go over 1 milligram. No need to. I'd also increase antioxidants as much as physically possible. Luckily both of these types of products are not very expensive.

Daily I'd be staying hydrated. I'd use enough salt. I'd take all 90 essential nutrients with extra selenium and antioxidants.

I'd seek to eat fermented foods and bone broth daily to further support a healthy digestive, and immune system. I'd buy a good juicer and start experimenting with many juices, adding in a bunch of my supplements to make it easier.

In my concoctions I would add a sea green. Spirulina and chlorella are cheap and I would buy bags of it.

I would add colloidal silver in. We haven't mentioned it much because there isn't that much to say. It is one of the strangest of the essential nutrients. We consider it essential, but it seems to have no metabolic role. It's not a cofactor or a building block or a spark plug like the other nutrients. It's not a hormone. It just seems to kill bad stuff inside and outside the body, selectively. It is said to support the immune system and promote healing, but we don't really know how.

I have a lot of great testimonials with colloidal silver. I know a guy who makes it in big jugs, he gets great results with people because they can afford to take so much at his price.

It will not turn you blue, by the way. That is a myth because it involves a silver salt, not colloidal silver. Obviously, if something turns you blue, you should stop taking it – not just continue taking it for years. Anyway, in goes a shot of colloidal silver to my daily drink.

It doesn't actually get that much more complicated than this. I would get serious about avoiding the bad foods, and serious about putting in as much of the good stuff as I could afford. But it's not an endless list. There are a few more things on it and we will get to them, but the rest of my focus for healing would simply be to stay positive and repeat this nutritional strategy every day.

I would remain calm and expect months of this discipline at least to really make the changes and heal the body. If I had a stressful job I would talk to my bosses. I would see if I could take some time off. Maybe I can work from home or reduce hours or workload.

Maybe I can have an assistant assigned to help get the important project done before I die. If it was an unpaid vacation offered I would see if I could take a loan to cover me a few months. I would ask family or friends if I needed it. I would at least tell them what I am trying to do and the type of help I could use. This is life or death, it's worth some sacrifice, in my opinion.

I have never faced cancer, but I have lived with pain. Knowing what I know now, there isn't much difference between the protocol for back pain and cancer. Both focus on loading the body up with nutrients and eliminating the problems. And the next biggest factor is stress.

I mentioned that circulation is likely to be involved in any cancer. I would say "all cancer includes a circulation problem", but I don't think I can back that up adequately in this type of a book. So I say its most likely the case. And so I would also do as many things that promote circulation as I could. Since my morning nutrient shake above only took a few minutes out of my day, and I'm well rested, I have the rest of the day to do *something* that encourages lymphatic movement, circulation, and low impact exercise.

Different types of massages, swinging on a swing, jumping on a trampoline or rebounder, even riding a roller coaster, all promote fluid movement in the body. You can feel it with the whooshing feeling going down the hill in a car or in a swing. All of these are useful and interchangeable. And there are treatments you can pay for which can promote circulation big time.

Professional massage, acupuncture, and cupping will be the most widely available therapies stimulating blood and lymph circulation. There are also machines available. A common one is called a shaker machine. It's a platform that shakes. More expensive models will have a wider range of functions, but they're all just different types or force of shaking. People with serious circulation issues will only be able to stand on the low rumble setting until they improve their circulation enough to tolerate higher vibration.

As they improve overall, they can increase the setting. This should be done multiple times a day. In our real life store in Windsor, Ontario, we have one of these machines. They are extremely useful, both for improving circulation, and for measuring the progress. Typically, within a few weeks a person can work their way up from a low rumble setting for a few minutes, to the strong firm vibration on the higher settings, for a longer time.

Some of these people can now walk again without pain. Some of these people were able to avoid limb amputation surgeries recommended by their physicians. Since blood sugar problems cause circulation problems, a result is limbs susceptible to gangrene, and eyes susceptible to blindness. These are circulation issues.

The shaker machine we have retails for around a thousand dollars. It can run 24/hrs a day, and the average person will get huge benefit by standing on it for only 20 minutes a day, just like a decent little low impact exercise session. This mimics much of the benefits of low impact exercise, without the exercise.

I'd also like to mention children. Sometimes we see children with cancers, but not often. They tend to go to cancer hospitals, not alternative people. But we see lots of kids with blood sugar problems. As I believe there is an immediate circulation problem whenever there is a blood sugar problem, I also believed that the circulation machines would be helpful for a kid with a blood sugar problem.

This thought process did not occur out of the kindness of my heart. I was dealing with a woman, sitting down at the table discussing her quite serious health problems. And her child was running around our store, knocking things off shelves and generally acting chaotically.

I called him over, asked him to try one of our pure colloidal mineral product samples. Then another, and another. Then I asked him to try the shaker machine. I put it on the highest setting, and he was completely glued to it. Staring straight ahead, with blank but focused attention, like someone had turned him off with his eyes still open. Small skinny kid, maybe 10 years old.

He stayed there and he stayed quiet and when he got off he said it felt really good, and his body was still tingling and still felt good. I began recommending it to children every time I had to talk serious-ly with their parents.

We also have something called a chi machine. It's a small box with two foot holsters. You lay down on a table or the floor, rest your feet in the holsters, and it sways back and forth in a steady rhyth-mic way until the timer stops it. It is extremely simple, and ex-tremely effective.

While doing it, it doesn't feel like much. Many civilians were clearly embarrassed to be laying on a massage table at our quack store, with legs swaying back and forth. At least we don't make them pay for it.

When the machine stops, a wave comes from the feet, up the body, like the feeling of getting off a small boat onto shore. If the person's circulation is fine, that wave will go all the way to the head, back down the body to the feet, and most or all of the way back up to the head. If their circulation is poor, the wave won't go very far.

As they do more sessions of about ten or twenty minutes each day if possible, they should quickly find the wave traveling farther up the body, until it is normal. At this point they should feel much better overall. This feeling of mechanical circulation stimulation can be quite addictive. It feels very good even when we have nothing wrong with us.

A chi machine costs about $50 on the low end and only a few hun-dred on the high end. These are not high-tech tools. One shakes, the other sways. If you can get to a park and ride the swings, that is free. You will get great benefit to do that with discipline, 20 or more minutes a day until you feel much better overall.

We have one more machine at our disposal I that should mention, because it's also deceptively simple. It's called a "neuro massage machine." It is names like this that make me understand why we are sometimes thought of as quacks. It is just a massage chair, a blindfold, and headphones that play relaxing sound sequences in tune with the massage. It's really relaxing, and that's all it is.

If you came to us in real life, we really don't have much in the form of emergency treatments. But sometimes people stumble into us in a state of near emergency. Our store is across the hall from a busy pharmacy and walk-in clinic. We had a lot of spillover. The clinic offered methadone treatment for drug addicts, and fentanyl for accident victims, so you can imagine that some real weird cases came from there.

Not really being equipped to handle a crisis, we're still willing to help. Sometimes the doctor in that walk-in kicked people out for being unruly. We'd literally be their last hope in their greatest time of need, and of course these people are the toughest type of people to deal with.

We offer a glass of very salty water. We offer some raw liquid plant derived minerals that are so strong they taste like mineral whiskey. If we are feeling generous, we can add more sophisticated supplements to the drink we offer.

We have a shaker machine, a chi machine, and a fancy relaxo chair. And we have people who swear that this short list of things helped them in an hour more than their doctors have helped them over a lifetime.

There are also people out there walking around who will swear to you that I changed their life only with a glass of salty water. Some of these people consider these experiences miracles, but I don't. These are all completely mechanical protocols.

I do have something to say that is closer to magic, and I am going to use this to lead into the next chapter on autoimmunity.

The list of things we have covered so far is most of the story, but there is more, and the first time it really made sense to me, was with lupus.

8. Autoimmune Diseases.

I am going to take a curveball approach to this chapter. And I am going to tell you this part of the story in more detail, or else you might not believe me.

Years ago we had a booth at a small health fair. It was at a large church in the small town I lived in. It was like a farmer's market with produce, but there were also various alternative health advocates there promoting all kinds of things. There were small honey farmers, yoga instructors promoting their businesses, and people like us selling packaged supplements and giving out information.

There were a few speakers inside, but I didn't see them because I was outside at the booth. Like most health fairs, it was pretty quiet, so I was talking with the other vendors and checking out their products and services. I like to hear the pitch, whatever it is. And vendors are great prospects for my business too.

To use the washrooms we had to go inside the church. To go inside, I was told that I could not bring in any device that had a signal turned on. If I wanted to go inside, I had to show that my phone had airplane mode turned on, data and WiFi signals turned off, or the whole phone off.

I had never been asked to do this before.

The explanation was that one of the speakers claimed to be extremely sensitive to electronic signals. He was there to give a talk about electronic frequencies and radiation. I decided I was going to speak to him after his talk.

Conveniently he came out to our booth and introduced himself. He used very simple language. He could feel the signals. It could be described as annoying or uncomfortable or even painful, which is why he requests a room free of it. But, he said, the real importance is long term. Whether you can feel it or not, it's there. And it could be affecting the body all the time.

He wasn't crazy, by my observation. He was straightforward and reasonable. I would call him a straight shooter. A bit kooky, but I probably am too.

I liked him and I enjoyed his story and for the first time I thought about invisible energy waves radiating from everything around me. I went home and looked out the window at the cell phone tower across the river, suddenly seeming ominous, yet I hadn't really noticed it before.

I never saw that guy again and I didn't do much research. I was busy with other things. But I began to pay more and more attention to electrical devices. I didn't know if I was playing tricks on myself, or whether I could really feel the computer mouse buzzing my hand.

I began to think that I was becoming more sensitive, just by paying attention. The buzz or hum of different devices around my apartment began to bother me. When the refrigerator was "running" I felt unease.

For a long time I told myself that I was making this up because I was expecting it. My increasing awareness didn't cause any pain or discomfort. In fact my pain and discomfort had almost entirely disappeared since I had started the nutrition program I was promoting. But it was more and more annoying.

I felt that I was pretty tolerant of difficult conditions. I have lived in very cold and very hot places. I have dealt with serious infections, I have conquered chronic pain, and I felt confident in traveling almost anywhere in the world by myself and with little money. The growing annoyance from the electronic devices seemed eventually to challenge my patience and resolve like no other challenge in life ever had.

Because I couldn't avoid it. Once I noticed it, it was everywhere around me. I felt paranoid and I knew that describing this whole thing would make me sound crazy. I didn't want the bed near a wall outlet. I didn't want to sit near a fridge, or an electric oven when it was running. I didn't want my phone in my pocket, or near my head.

I had never been particularly picky about music quality. I cared whether I liked the music or not. My father was an audio technician and a musician, so maybe I picked up some things, but until this point in my life I was content to listen to the music I liked on any device that was convenient.

As I became more sensitive to frequencies in general, I found that digital music began to sound "off." Flat and lifeless, like distilled water without salt. Sometimes it sounded offensive. I liked the music, but not the sound. My favorite music didn't sound right on the computer or mp3 or CD. It sounded fine on my analog vinyl system.

Somewhere in this time I was visiting my mother. At the local flea market, I saw that one of the vendors had a product from the company I was promoting. I stopped to talk to him about it. He was an enthusiastic distributor as well, but that was not what his booth was about.

He asked if he could try a demonstration with me, and we did. He proved to me that my balance was terrible in general, and that it was even worse with a phone in my hand. I couldn't argue with it.

Then he put a magic disc on a cheap nylon strap on my wrist, and did the test again. He was twice my age and easily twice my strength, but with the magic disc and the same test as before, my balance and strength was incredibly enhanced against his force.

My first skeptical instinct was that he might have been yanking my arm out sideways on the first tests, making me look very easily toppled. If he aimed straight down on the next test with the magic disc, then I should appear much stronger.

But it was no trick. My girlfriend was there watching, we did it multiple times, and quite honestly, I trusted the guy as soon as we started talking. I felt he was hard headed but genuine. I felt he really believed in his magic bracelets.

I didn't buy anything from him.

Back at my mother's house, she told me that someone was renting her garage for storage. There was a car, and a bunch of other stuff in there. I didn't think anything of it.

It turned out that that guy renting the garage was the same guy at the flea market selling the magic bracelets. His name is Mike. The stuff in the garage was his summer car and all his stuff behind the flea market business.

I called him, and he came by the house. We introduced each other more formally, shook hands, and he made me a steel bracelet with two magic discs attached, as a gift. Right there on the driveway.

I didn't feel much when I put it on. And I also wasn't paying that much attention. We were in town for some event, and we were on the move. I kept the bracelet on and we went back to our little town.

Soon after, my girlfriend at the time had her wisdom teeth taken out. She was in bed with swollen chipmunk cheeks, in a drugged stupor, and I thought that letting her wear my magic bracelet might help her a bit. She saw the demonstration and was just as impressed and puzzled as I was. You hear of carnival trick quacks at flea markets, but you really don't often encounter them.

I gave her my bracelet and the moment I took it off, it felt like I had taken the battery out of my back. It felt like my body was telling me directly: "put it back on." I didn't have a lot of money at the time, but I called Mike and asked if he could give me a deal on another bracelet. He did. I have worn one since.

Until this point, I can't recall really believing that fate had much to do with the turn of events. But meeting Mike would end up being very important to my path in the alternative health world, and this will bring us to why we are talking about this when we're supposed to be talking about autoimmunity.

Back in my little town, that girl and I had broken up, and I was in a sort of despair in an empty apartment, in an end-of-the-road type of town that I had no roots in, and I didn't know what I was going to do next.

I don't remember if Mike called me or I called him, but I remember standing there in my empty living room, looking out across that nice little river, and at that ominous cell phone tower, as Mike told me bluntly: "I'm out of this place man. I can't take all the hassle out here in [east Toronto], all the traffic, all the stress."

He said he was moving to Windsor, Ontario, a small industrial city across the river from Detroit, Michigan. His daughter lived there and he had a location picked out to open a store under the same guise as his booth at the market.

He didn't ask if I wanted to join. He didn't know my situation. But my lease was coming up, and I didn't want to pay for the place anyway. I told him I'd pack up and go with him.

At this point, I still didn't really know anything about electromagnetic frequencies (EMF), and I really didn't know much about the magic discs either. I was still rooted in nutrition and I was there to help him sell all the different things he had, including our supplements.

Since I had really only seen his demonstration once (when he did it on me), I hadn't had much exposure to his process. And since I wasn't at the market long, I hadn't really heard the entire pitch. When we met we mostly talked business or talked shop. We had even been on the radio together at some time along here, and we still hadn't heard each other out entirely. But now I got to hear the entire sales process, and I had a lot of questions.

Mike kept mentioning testimonials for health problems that I was taught were entirely nutritional. My head was already spinning about this, and I had already begun going through a bunch of books on radiation to catch myself up, when one day at work Mike mentioned one of his testimonials about lupus.

I really had to step back and sit down. Most of the claims he was making were about physical problems, and I still had a lot of questions about that. But the symptoms of lupus are mostly digestive. Blood sugar problems, circulatory problems, and a low-grade allergic type of experience in the body is the basic description of a lupus patient. Inflammation all over, basically.

The guy he was talking about was on video giving his testimonial, but as usual, Mike said his real off-camera testimony is even more amazing. Long story short, he felt a lot better extremely quickly, credited to a frequency tuning disc. But this is lupus. He didn't do any nutritional changes. I didn't understand.

Mike is more of a mechanic than a technician, so he wasn't really able to explain it either. But he was able to tell me that he has other similar cases, so-called autoimmune patients who felt much better in many ways, very quickly, with the addition of the magic discs.

As I dug into this one case, trying to justify an explanation as to how this person could achieve this result with an anti-radiation device, I had a few realizations.

The first usual suspect is placebo. It really is an awesome healing tool. But this seemed too dramatic. The guy was very overweight, very obviously experiencing serious digestive issues, and circulation issues. His cheeks were red with "spider web" patterns, typical of lupus. He looked like he was having a low-grade allergic reaction, typical of lupus, and he reported that this was constant for him, as expected.

I have to reserve the power of belief as a factor in any major transformation. And I expect that strong hope that something will work, and desire for it to work, will greatly enhance the benefit they experience. But I was not willing to credit belief with this transformation. I had been around the healing business just enough to have dealt with a few "autoimmune" people by that point. I knew that they were tough cases. They had to change their eating habits, they had to put in a bunch of nutrients, and this has to take time. Cells don't regenerate overnight. Healing and digestive strategies take time. It just shouldn't be possible to turn this around in minutes like they were all claiming.

When I first met Mike back at the flea market, the first real question he asked me was if I had any pain. This was part of his process. Often, the person did have a pain, and they could point to at least one chronically painful spot somewhere on their body. Mike's strategy was to tape a disc to that spot immediately, and then carry on with answering their questions about his "Live Pain Free!" banner, and he would be moving toward doing the demonstration as well.

He did this because he knew it was likely that the pain would disappear in the time they were talking. He would bet that in the few minutes he had with the average person, that in that time he could eliminate at least one pain. This is an amazing thing when you think about it. We are not taught about this type of thing in nutrition.

With nutrition I expect results, but not immediately. In a few minutes I can barely expect to make a proposal and a transaction, let alone a result. They have to take action and continue for the expected "feel better" part of the deal. If there was a five-minute method, it felt like we were wrong about nutrition.

There was an explanation right in front of me. It was in the books, and it was in my life. I knew people who did "live blood analysis." They look at blood in real time, "live." I knew that blood cells could crinkle up and clump together under many forms of stress.

It suddenly made sense. All this nutrient stuff I was taught about was transported in the blood. Digestive problems could cause blood problems, we call this "dirty blood", or "sticky blood." This is basically "leaky gut", undigested food particles getting into the blood via the intestines.

The blood correctly responds to these foreign food particles, supposed to have been broken down further and chemically altered in the digestive process before being absorbed. The blood clots attention around these undigested food particles and this causes an overall congestion problem in the blood. Like white blood cells attacking a sickness, the bodies of cells and pathogens add up to a mucous we call dirty blood. It is almost like an allergic reaction, or the body responding to a virus.

That's one way to have compromised blood. Another is to have a nutrient deficiency severe enough to affect the blood. The body will take nutrients from virtually every system in the body before it messes with the blood. A problem in the blood is a huge problem. If there's not enough of the right stuff for blood to function properly, the body will fail catastrophically. Every blood deficiency has a disease named after it.

But even under good conditions, when there is no digestive problem, no dirty blood problem, and the person is supplementing with all of the essential nutrients in optimum amounts, we can see in live blood analysis that healthy blood can crumple up, stick together, slow down, and look visibly terrible compared to healthy blood relieved of the stress.

This was it, that is the answer. If radiation can affect the blood, and we know it does because live blood analysis shows this, then all of the nutrients, oxygen, sugar, and waste products that the blood needs to transport around can be compromised by this.

Electronic devices have increased in use to the point where "everyone" has something on them or near them sending signals and attempting to receive them. The fields are invisible but they are all around us. Voltage traveling through wires has increased significantly over the decades. All of this is a more stressful environment for us to operate in. It affects our blood cells, and they are responsible for transporting every other important thing you can name in and out of the body.[xviii]

If someone's blood is fully impacted by this radiation stress, then relieving that stress alone can show a near-miraculous result very quickly.

The discs aren't magic, and they have a mechanical explanation. But I wasn't satisfied with the explanation Mike gave for the relief of symptoms. He said the discs were charged with frequencies. The same frequencies as our bones, nervous system, and muscular system. This is assumed to enhance our own energy fields, protecting against harmful ones. He had some lines memorized by Nikola Tesla about frequencies, and he focused on the demonstrations and whether someone stopped shaking or felt pain relief as the conversation happened.

I also saw him bet, many times, that letting someone take a sample bracelet home for the night would bring them back for a purchase. Not only did most of them come back and return the sample, most of them also bought a steel bracelet with the discs installed. Many of them remained highly skeptical, but continued to wear the discs.

I was used to standing beside doctors and professionals and talking seriously about health with people who are in serious condition. I am used to having solid mechanical answers for them. I was not comfortable pitching magic discs that relieve pain just because of magic energy. But now I had a mechanical explanation: relieving the blood.

I stayed in that town long enough to see many hundreds of demonstrations, witness and meet many testimonials, and do many demonstrations myself. Many people tried to fool the discs, but they couldn't. They work under a steel-toed boot, they work if you slip it into someone's pocket and don't tell them, they work on dogs and cats having mobility trouble in old age.

I don't think a dog has any expectation or placebo response to a frequency tuning disc. If they had serious trouble going up the stairs, or had lost that ability, and then can quite suddenly go up them with ease, something has changed. Dogs, like people, require time to heal injuries and rebuild tissues. But they can also be impacted by the radiation in our homes and our modern world.

The point of this long divergence, is that my time in this part of the alternative health business (the anti-radiation world), gave me everything I felt I needed to finally understand health problems in our society and what to do about them.

In my time with the discs I have heard and seen things I know make us sound like liars for saying. I have seen people stand up from wheelchairs, who were nearly completely immobile moments before. I have met people who walked into our store with crutches, and walked out on their own two feet. We have had people with many varieties of cancers and autoimmune diseases report incredible turnarounds.

Most of these people did not buy our nutrition products. Most of them did not change their lifestyles. These are regular people, most of whom have lived in that blue-collar town their whole lives. In any case, it's a lot easier to sell a magic bracelet than it is a healthy lifestyle, as it is a one-time purchase, not an ongoing commitment.

This brings me back to what I think is the main difference between cancer and an immune problem. As far as I can tell, cancer is what happens when a catastrophically compromised body fails big time in one system of the body. The liver is dying, they call it liver cancer. The skin is messed up, they call it skin cancer. It's a growth in the brain, it's brain cancer. Growth in the prostate, prostate cancer.

We've seen many things that can contribute to system failures. Digestive problems can lead to nutrient deficiencies and dirty blood and blood sugar problems and circulation problems. Nutrient deficiencies can exist without a digestive problem, just by not having enough nutrients in the diet.

Those nutrients are responsible for every system in the body, so if there's not enough, there's a problem somewhere in the body. Selenium also happens to be one of those key nutrients involved in both the liver and prostate, by the way. No coincidence.

We've seen that stress of all kinds can impact the basic ability of the body to maintain and repair itself, and we've added electronic frequencies to that list of possible stresses on the body.

So when it happens in an identifiable system, and the allopathic professions don't have an explanation, they call it a cancer. When the body is failing in multiple systems, or is a general immune problem, I believe, they call it an autoimmune disease.

Now, there is a complicated aspect here having to do with antibodies. We're going to talk more about "blood markers", which is what I prefer to call them, in the next chapter on AIDS.

For now, it is worth pointing out that there is no agreed explanation about autoimmunity in the mainstream medical world. They say blood marker antibodies have something to do with it, but not one of their so-called autoimmune diseases have a consistent correlation between the presence of antibodies and the presence of symptoms.

This means that some people who have symptoms called an autoimmune disease don't have the appropriate expected blood markers. And some people without symptoms have these markers.

To me, this means there is not a correlation. But this is what tests for these diseases are about.

We don't need a test to see that autoimmune patients have a problem. By our questionnaire or by looking at them we can easily see multiple problems in the body.[xix]

In my experience, there is always bad food involved. Always. There is always a food causing an inflammatory reaction. Even the guy who got the great result quickly, was still eating the wrong foods and will still have corresponding health problems. At least he feels better.

If a body is failing, there is always a nutrient deficiency involved. The body needs nutrients to heal. If it feels bad it needs more nutrients.

Chances are, the person with an "autoimmune disease" is on a pharmaceutical drug. The way these drugs are marketed, they say these drugs suppress the immune system, under the assumption that the immune system is attacking itself.

We do not believe the immune system attacks itself. We believe there is likely many separate problems going on in the body. Food is probably one. Nutrient deficiency is definitely one. EMF stress can most definitely be another. Our intention is to support the immune system, rather than oppress it. If the body can heal itself, then we want to support that.

I took this tangent because we were in the middle of listing everything I would do if I found out I had cancer. I would get strict on my eating, get serious on my supplementing, I would encourage circulation and low impact exercise and seek a lot of rest and relaxation.

But I would also get serious about reducing the radiation around me. I would wear a frequency tuning disc bracelet. Unlike nutrition, which must be consumed every day more or less, a device can be purchased once, and they can be collected. I wear one on the wrist and one on the ankle and I don't think I'm going to stop that.

I've also now lived far from cities. I've been out in the desert with my shoes off grounded to the Earth. I've taken the bracelet off and *still* felt weaker without it. So I do believe it has an enhancement effect on its own. And I do believe that it is one of the things we should definitely do to reduce the stress of EMF on our body.

That's only one device, but it's the cheapest one that actually works, in my experience.

There are a few key things that can reduce our exposure. The biggest source for most people these days will be the phone in their hand or pocket. There are devices that can reduce the fields of the phone. I use one, and I don't like to use devices without one.[xx] The cheap ones on the market don't work well enough, or at all, in my opinion.

But even with that, I don't put the phone in my pocket. Basically ever. Maybe 10 minutes in a year, the odd time I have my hands full. The phone never goes to my head. I speak with headphones attached by a wire, or on speakerphone.

I also don't pay a phone bill, so airplane mode can always be on. Everyone I know and do business with can contact me through a number of different apps, but not by phone number.

This is not for everyone, I guess, but I find it great. I pay for home internet by a cable, and most of my phone time I plug the phone into an Ethernet adapter. I do use WiFi, and I can run my online business on my phone through Ethernet cables or WiFi, or my wire-connected computer. When I go outside, I have peace. The data signal on my phone can be turned off all the time. The Bluetooth is off. It's the best I can do for now. I do travel frequently and yet I have operated without a phone bill for several years now, and I encourage it.

WiFi is also EMF, but it's not as bad as having it in your pocket or at your temple. You can make or buy a Faraday cage that will reduce the output of your WiFi router. In many cases you can get a smaller router and it will work fine.

You can shield some of the bigger sources with any type of metal plate or foil. Yes, foil. Don't seal off the whole house, and you don't need to wear it on your head, though it would offer some protection. Many people are making silver fabric clothing, including hats, for this reason. They also make EMF-shielding paint, with metal in it. In my house, I foiled the wall behind the smart meter and put a bookshelf in front of that.

The refrigerator will be one of the larger sources in the house. If your favorite chair shares a wall with the fridge, I'd shield that wall. If I lived next to a cell phone tower, an electrical transfer station, high voltage power lines, or above a subway, I would move. There isn't a way to completely shield yourself from extremely strong sources close by.

This is pretty much the last major category of the alternative health world: energy, frequencies, and self-healing in the countryside.

The people I had heard who had chronic illness or a serious diagnosis, and basically went home to die, typically left a city and went home to the countryside. Away from much of the radiation.

The extended fishing trip is away from all the electro stress in the atmosphere, the constant buzz. The meditation trip is peaceful in part because of this. The singing bowls and tuning forks and grounding blankets, if they help, I would say it was because those frequencies helped relieve some of the ongoing EMF stress temporarily.

I am also willing to connect juicing to this. I've already mentioned a few reasons why juicing might help someone feel better, but here is two steps deeper. Minerals are inorganic in most of the world. That means they're rocks, or sand, or shells. In sea water all the minerals are present in trace amounts, but not in organic form.

When a plant absorbs a mineral, it converts the inorganic mineral into a charged electrical form, sometimes called "organic minerals", "ionic", "fulvic", "humic", or "colloidal." We call them colloidal and promote them with this explanation.

In soils, this process requires bacteria and fungus in the soil to participate in the acceptance of the mineral into the root of the plant.[xxi] The microorganisms in the soil essentially "predigest" the minerals for absorption into the plant. These are my simple words for a very complicated process. Sea water is full of microorganisms already, and they also facilitate the process in sea plants.

These colloidal minerals are interesting and I'm going to hover here for a moment. If you take a handful of sand or dirt or any inorganic minerals, and you add them to water, they will sink to the bottom after some time.

If you shake it all up, it will become cloudy, and then eventually it will settle again. Colloidal minerals have many interesting properties, but the most interesting to me is that colloidal minerals do not settle. The explanation is that they are electrically charged (ionic), and so they remain in suspension indefinitely because they remain repelled from each other electrically. Fascinating, really. It is like perpetual motion, or magnetism. Like a refrigerator magnet staying stuck perpetually, the particles remain there charged, apparently forever.

I mentioned magic earlier, well this is the real magic as far as I'm concerned. Not only are organic colloidal mineral particles much smaller than inorganic forms, the plant-derived colloidal forms also seem to be required for optimal structure and function and longevity, while inorganic minerals are difficult to absorb and many of them can be harmful.

Arsenic is an agreed upon essential mineral for all vertebrates. All animals with a spine. But it can kill in the inorganic form. Same story with pretty much every element on the list. It can be essential, and it can kill you in the wrong form or dose.

So plants, through plant magic, convert the earth into an interesting electrical form of energetic nutrition, and that's interesting. But they also change the structure of the water. Structured water is another huge topic that deserves detail but must be included briefly because this is a long list.

In my attempt to give a proper summary of the many options available for getting closer to health, structured water has to be mentioned. Clean water is important, but structure seems much more important.

In nature, stagnant water is bad. We don't want to drink it. We have to do something with it. Boil it, maybe capture the steam. Maybe add salt or other things like medicinal tea leaves, in the hopes of avoiding plagues that can come from bad water.

Running water is much cleaner. Water running over rocks creates vortex patterns, spirals, which seem to clean and structure the water. Ocean water also has its own structure. This is the structure used for the product I am most familiar with.

There are spiral taps sold as water structure devices. I believe they do help. I believe the water is better if it runs through a vortex before you consume it. There are also receptacles marketed to be shaped so as to not allow the water to settle, encouraging a healthier structure.

I do know all of this can sound loony, which is why I included it all in this weird chapter. I'll give one more thought on this before we get back to juicing.

At one point in my life I worked in a chemistry lab analyzing sea water samples. There can be many steps involved in preparing samples, adding reactive agents (reagents), letting them sit on timers, heating them, or cooling them, etc.

Some tests require that you spin the sample in a vortex. Measuring chlorophyll, for example, each sample had to be spun on a vortex or it would screw up the results. It would measure low. I thought that was very interesting at the time, but I didn't really get it.

Since then, I started stirring whatever I was drinking, in a quick vortex, before I drank it. It seems to change the taste of almost anything you drink if you pay attention to it.

So why is juicing so effective? On top of being an easy to digest, nutritionally dense drink that is easy to add even more supplements to, it is typically spun in a vortex before serving, but even better is the fact that the water was already structured inside of the plant.

Plant juice is structured water. Celery juicing every day for 90 days is one of the most popular alternative health trends of our current time. This is structured water. We can't eat enough plants to really get this benefit. Most of the liquid we would be consuming throughout the day will be from a tap or bottle or something other than a plant.

It takes a lot of oranges to make a glass of orange juice. But that is structured water.

We are mostly water.

Water is a necessary cofactor for most or all processes in the body. Water is the substrate in which all the chemical processes in the body take place.

In the health business, there's a saying to sell water filters: "If you don't have a water filter, you are the filter."

Wow. It sold me. Filter for life.

So clean water is important. The structure of water is important. We are mostly water. And structured water seems to be good for us.

Since we are mostly water, this is most of our energy field, if I have come far enough to use language like this. When we enhance our own water system with properly structured water, we are enhanced dramatically.

And I mean really dramatically. I mean a structured water program can rebound someone's health just as well as any other miracle I've witnessed. And juicing is one way to do it.

It's an expensive way to do it, but nonetheless.

This is protection from stress to our own energy field, signified by the blood. This is witnessed by live blood analysis. Many structured water products use live blood analysis to pitch their water. The blood can be seen to be relieved in real time.

To wrap up this segment, I want to be clear that I am not saying radiation is the cause of all autoimmune diseases. EMF is one factor that contributes to an unhealthy body, and some people are sensitive enough where nothing else will work if they don't address the EMF in their lives. Bad foods and nutrient deficiencies are practically guaranteed to be involved in any problem labeled "autoimmune", and not everyone that I have seen eliminate these symptoms has addressed EMF. But the real amazing thing to me is the people who did nothing *except* address the EMF, and turned their health around.

We covered rheumatoid arthritis already, the oddball in the arthritis group and in the autoimmune group. Our explanation is that the rheumatoid component is caused by a bug infection. The arthritis part is partially damage from the bug, and degeneration from nutrient deficiency. This barely has anything to do with the immune system, other than the assumption that the immune system is trying to fight the infection.

The other autoimmune diseases are not as clear as this. They're not clear at all. The antibody explanation isn't clear at all. The mainstream treatments are not successful at all. The drugs they prescribe people can do serious damage or kill them. The symptoms of autoimmune problems are generalized throughout the body, usually in the form of susceptibility to illness and basic obvious digestive problems and nutrient deficiencies.

After years of trying to figure out how antibodies are actually correlated with disease, and what they actually are, I am convinced that I do not understand antibodies. I have given up because I am convinced that no one else truly understands them either.

But I know for certain that everyone being told they have an autoimmune problem, has many problems. One could be more of a problem than others. I have heard so many people claim total transformation just by quitting gluten, or grains altogether, I cannot count them all.[xxii]

It could just be gluten, it could just be catastrophic nutrient deficiency, it could be hyper stress from life, or hyper sensitivity to radiation stress. More likely is a combination of most or all of these things. Maybe other stresses too. Maybe the cat wakes them up every night in the middle of the night and they haven't slept all the way through the night in years as a result. Maybe the kids are trouble makers and they're losing their hair from that on top of every-thing. In the public market we hear about all kinds of stresses.[xxiii]

An ongoing infection problem could be a big factor that was over-looked. A fungal infection of some form is likely in everyone I've ever seen with an autoimmune problem other than rheumatoid. But even with rheumatoid, many of them are likely to have a fungal infection problem as well. An immune problem encourages growth of all the bad stuff.

All of these stresses can contribute, and relieving any one of them could feel like a magic bullet for the person experiencing the relief.

We recommend approaching health generally. We don't "treat" au-toimmunity because, well we don't even believe the term makes sense, but we also don't even need to target the problem. We need to use every strategy we can to promote a healthy body. Eliminat-ing the bad stuff, adding the good stuff at appropriate doses, and recognizing that electrical frequencies could be interfering with all of it, by design of modern life.

There is more we can do to promote relief from radiation stress, and they are also healing techniques on their own.

For centuries people have left cities on healing trips to the country-side. Some of them left cities because of lung problems, and felt the air was cleaner in the country, which is true. Many of them had general pain problems, arthritis, lack of hunger, all kinds of things, and they thought they'd feel better in the country, or were given ad-vice from a doctor to go to the countryside. There have always been many theories on why this could be beneficial. When people went out to the country, they tended to go to a cottage or a manor or a mountain or a beach.

Any of these gets us away from the psychological stress of the city, but some of these we believe to be healing in themselves. The beach is full of "negative ions." It is said that the "bad energy" associated with EMF is "positive ions." So negative beats positive. I think they should have named them the other way around, but hey.

The air around the ocean and beach are said to be loaded with these negative ions, combating the bad ions or enhancing us or however we choose to describe it. I don't think we really need to understand it. The beach has good energy. So that appears to promote rest, relaxation, and healing. Running water has good energy, and that appears to encourage good health as well.

Salt lamps, said to "reduce EMF stress in the house", also stream negative ions into the air. I find them highly beneficial.

Mountains are big rocks. Rocks have good energy. I live in a place called the Canadian Shield. It's a gigantic rock. You put the shovel in the ground, and very soon you hit rock. And it stretches down to parts of America as well. The energy side of the alternative health world is much closer to the hippy end of things than I am used to in the nutrition end. We really are talking about energy in rocks here, but I'm serious about it. We also talk as if the cells of trees act like the frequency tuning discs, charged with good energy that radiates negative ions.

When I first went way up north, I couldn't understand why I got so tired in the forest. On this gigantic rock, surrounded by trees in every direction, I felt like I was being waved to sleep. I wanted to sleep all day. This is very unusual for me, as I had had trouble sleeping my whole life.

I believe this is the healing energy at work and I believe it is necessary to know about. It is a much healthier environment – nature stuff – as far as I can tell, than any indoor therapeutic environment. Nature can heal, I believe. The body asking for sleep is doing it for a reason. To become excessively relaxed and tired in the middle of the day is probably the result of something therapeutic.

If you look, you will find many people who embraced a "natural" lifestyle, in as many different ways as possible. Something as little as spending time with the feet grounded on the Earth can go a long way. Implementing awareness of electrical pollution can go a long way. Trips out to nature can be phenomenally restorative, for both body and mind.

I didn't want to reiterate the *Fake Diseases* theory here because I think you get it by this point. None of the so-called autoimmune diseases can really be diseases if they are the result of mechanical problems in the body. Though there is a reasonably long list of possible mechanical problems, we have covered most of them. Doctors get away with labeling autoimmune problems as diseases because they seem to want to treat them. But they don't know how to. Helping a person get better from any of the symptoms on the list of the average autoimmune problem has nothing to do with the toolkit of the allopathic professional.

There is nothing to cut out when it comes to an autoimmune problem. There are no useful surgical interventions. There are no drugs that support and promote the body's natural ability to heal itself. And some of the foods on the "food plate", we're saying, can screw up the body big time – enough to look like an "autoimmune disease."

It is up to us who we take our health problems to. Knowing all of this, I wouldn't go to a medical doctor if I had this type of problem. And I wouldn't bother calling it a disease. It is not transmitted, it is multidimensional. And none of the routes to real relief are medicinal. Maybe a medicine can help them, but it's not a cure.

If syphilis is a disease because it requires treatment by a licensed practitioner, then autoimmune problems, cancer, digestive disorders, blood sugar problems, bone and joint problems, and birth defects, should not be called diseases.

Knowing all of this, we can tackle the final topics.

9. AIDS.

Initially I wanted to start this book with AIDS. AIDS is, I think, the best true example of a fake disease.

I have used the word *fake* kind of loosely in this book. Most of the stuff we've covered so far is absolutely real. Birth defects are real, bone, blood sugar, and digestive problems are real. Cancer and autoimmune diseases, while poorly defined, are still experiences that require a name.

My problem so far has mostly just been that many things shouldn't be called diseases. The title of a disease is mostly misleading. The legal appropriation of the word disease is necessary to properly categorize things that require treatment from regulated professionals. Most of our list does not meet this criteria, and so should not be thought of as disease.

Most of what we talked about can be easily prevented and reversed. That's important and empowering. But how do we protect ourselves from a disease that doesn't exist at all?

Syphilis is a disease because it requires treatment. Technically it's an infection, but legally it's a disease. I prefer to use the correct technical language to describe specific things. A spade is most usefully referred to as a spade, and an infection is most usefully referred to as an infection. I'm totally okay with syphilis being classified as a disease, even if it doesn't help our understanding of the problem. All infections should fall under the legal umbrella of professions equipped to deal with infections. The market should be protected from false claims about real diseases. This is a big part of the point in the legal terminology. Classifying something as a disease not only determines who can treat it, but also what we can all say about it.

None of us can go on TV and talk directly about a cure for cancer. With the mainstream understanding of cancer, or the one we have covered here, it is not appropriate to talk this way, and this is legally important in the modern world.

I believe in the free market and that people should be able to make their own informed decisions. But if we *do* have medical regulations, they might as well be used to set the appropriate boundaries for talking about medical things. This isn't censorship as much as it is agreeing what words mean. Agreeing what words mean is part of the foundation of law. Disease, treatment, and cure, are serious legal words.

If disease can mean any health issue, we will have a problem unless we are equipped to deal with health issues. If health issues must be treated, we must go to a doctor. If a doctor can't help, we still have an issue. If they make it worse, you get the idea. So that's my problem with calling chronic illness, chronic pain, birth defects, and body failure "disease."

My bigger problem is in completely made up diseases.

Syphilis is an infection. It infects us, we show symptoms, we take drug, drug kills bug, infection is over. Infections can be cured.

AIDS is supposedly caused by an infection with "HIV", a supposed virus. I say "supposed", because there is no absolute proof that a virus causes the problem, and there is no absolute proof that what we call "AIDS" is even real. They say there are two strains of *Lentivirus* that can cause AIDS. If the supposedly HIV "infected" person "gets worse" beyond the arbitrary limit, they now say they have AIDS.

So AIDS is the name for the HIV patient in poor condition. Syphilis is killed with a drug, but the H viruses are not. HIV, HSV, HPV, and dare I say, even hepatitis (A, B, or C), are incredibly ambiguous "diseases", and I am not sure if any of them are real. Anti viral pharmaceuticals have terribly unpredictable results with the H's.

There are a lot of people out there now claiming that "terrain theory" explains all "viruses." I think they have a lot of good points. Viruses are all around us, inside of us, everywhere all of the time. Bacteria and other potentially dangerous "pathogens" are also around us all the time. The only major difference is bacteria, fungus, worms and so on all have cells, while viruses apparently do not.

It is quite easy to *know* that we have been infected by a bug. It turns out to be quite a bit more difficult to prove an infection by a virus.

It is even more difficult to prove beyond confusion that a therapy actually works against a virus.

The single most effective treatment for virus "infection" is grandma's recipe – rest, heat, liquids, and time. I feel like keeping the quotations around *infection* when talking about viruses, because it does not seem to be clear that AIDS is actually an infection.

The same problem exists for antibodies. I have many problems with the way testing is done in the first place. The guy who invented the PCR test, Kary Mullis, also publicly doubted the efficacy of the test in use for disease diagnosis. Nonetheless, even if the tests were 100% accurate, we still have many left over questions about the unpredictability of blood markers.

People can still carry blood markers long after any sign of an "infection" with an H virus has vanished. This is not the case with bacterial infections. If you beat a bug, it's gone. But "infection" with an H virus seems to be able to affect us forever.

Most people infected with any virus, usually a flu of some kind, tend to "get better" with time, regardless of the course of action. If time passes, they are likely to get better, with or without medicine. Most honest doctors will answer about viruses the same way we do – if you've already got symptoms, there's not much you can do, it has to pass.

Very few compounds will speed up this process. We can support the body's ability to defend itself and give it more nutrition. This might ease our misery, but the sickness will still need time to clear. Usually around 2 weeks, more or less. Kids, adults, elderly, all need time.

This is not true for syphilis. If you leave it, you will get worse and worse until it becomes life threatening. If you still do nothing, you will probably die from the infection. Actually this isn't completely true. We have probably all heard of the "Tuskegee experiment", where the United States Public Health Service and the CDC left a group of 399 men with syphilis untreated. This is commonly used as an example of the big bad government, and I agree that it is a highly unpalatable part of our history. But what isn't often mentioned is that several of those untreated men lived with the syphilis for a full and long life. One of them, Ernest Hendon, lived to age 96, which is much more than the American life expectancy during those decades.

Even though I've used syphilis throughout this book as a classic example of a real qualified disease, it isn't completely clear that syphilis is life-threatening unless there are other factors contributing to an unhealthy body. Mr. Hendon must have done several other things right, including getting enough minerals and vitamins to be healthy, and avoiding some or all of the foods on our bad list – I assume he still put his wood ashes in the garden, or consumed them directly, getting his plant derived minerals, and since he remained untreated for his syphilis, I assume he also avoided other medical "treatment", which is a good thing to do if you want to avoid death by medication or surgery.

A blood sugar problem will not go away by accident, something needs to change. Aches and pains and rashes can come and go, but chances are the frequency of appearance will not change much unless the lifestyle is changed.

By this one factor, time, we see that viral infections are different in at least one important way from all of the other diseases we have seen. No matter what the PCR test says, if we give it time, we are not likely to suffer long term. It's a bit weird to think of it this way, because AIDS is only promoted with fear. But all symptoms related to viruses do seem to pass, if they don't kill us.

I am very doubtful that viruses, at least retroviruses, "infect" us in anything close to the same way as a bacterium or worm or fungus. We are told that viruses use our cells to host their DNA, but everywhere else we look on Earth, we see viruses. Animals can fail rapidly like humans under bad conditions. They can appear to be suffering from viral type illnesses too. But the terrain theory holds that this possibility is always there. If we become too far from "healthy", we are susceptible to begin looking diseased.

It's not easy to prove a negative. But they have also sold us this disease without proper proof, in my opinion. The test they use to look for markers of this disease is questioned by many of the people involved with creating it, including the main guy who got the Nobel Prize for it. I expect that he understands the test better than I do, and he says it's bogus, in my translation.

I am not the only one who has doubted that HIV/AIDS is an infection. In 1993 Dr. Robert Willner famously injected himself with HIV "infected" blood, multiple times in multiple cities. He said that most AIDS deaths were actually caused by the immune-suppressing drug AZT, which was the main "treatment" for AIDS. He wrote a whole book about it called *Deadly Decption: The Proof That Sex and HIV Absolutely Do Not Cause AIDS.*

The controversies behind PCR and false positives could be a book itself. But to have a disease on a spectrum based on markers that are only found by a dodgy test, does not give me the confidence to call this a disease or an infection at all.

The word "spectrum" is important. Syphilis is not a spectrum. You have it, or you do not have it. No in-between. No partial syphilis. No "just a little bit" of syphilis. No "you still have the syphilis, but your markers are low." None of this would make sense for syphilis because syphilis is an infection.

What kind of infection operates on a spectrum? Excellent question.

A fake infection, is my speculative answer.

The huge majority of adults in the western world will have PCR blood markers for "herpes." They call this HSV. In my opinion, all the H's are the same, in that they are not infections. If the word "infection" is used to describe syphilis, then it cannot be used to describe any of the H retroviruses. The HIV, HSV, HPV so-called infections do not match the appearance of other viral infections.

I want to include hepatitis here as well because the symptoms of this supposed infection are remarkably indistinct – they are symptoms you could have with any general "sickness." Many of us have probably had these symptoms when we had to stay home from school as kids, probably from the common flu. Symptoms of hepatitis include: fever, fatigue, loss of appetite, nausea, vomiting, abdominal pain, dark urine (dehydration), light-colored stools, joint pain, and jaundice. Jaundice is the most serious thing on this list, and jaundice is a nutrient problem – caused by a digestive problem, or vitamin deficiencies, probably caused by the sickness itself.

They say these symptoms can appear 2-6 months after "infection." They also want us to get vaccinated against this mysterious thing. But they tell us that the risk factors for hepatitis are pretty much the same as HIV: male on male sex, intravenous drug use, people who already "have" HIV, people who have had sex with someone else "with" hepatitis, people "requiring" immunosuppressive "therapy"[4], people with severe kidney disease, etc. So if you already have a serious problem (kidney disease, or something "requiring" immunosuppressive "therapy") then you might show these generalized signs of bad health. This only makes me think: Duh. If you're unhealthy, you might show other signs of being unhealthy. How is this a specific disease?

The majority of adults in the western world supposedly have markers for herpes in their blood. But the majority of adults in the western world do not show symptoms of herpes. HSV is the name below an arbitrary threshold, and herpes is what it's called when there's symptoms. Symptoms tend to occur when there are more markers in the blood. So herpes is to HSV what AIDS is to HIV.

Even the mainstream medical world seems to believe that you have

---

4   I know all the quotes are obnoxious, but I have a very hard time repeating
    these words as simple facts.

to be *unhealthy* for any symptoms of HSV to appear. Having blood markers present is not enough to be called "herpes." You can supposedly "have" the "disease" without having symptoms. So are the symptoms a result of an infection or the result of an unhealthy body?

It seems quite clear that the symptoms of HSV, HPV, HIV, and hepatitis (A, B, or C), are a result of an unhealthy body. Terrain theory. Don't believe me? First, go get a test for herpes. It's a safe bet that you'll have antibodies. If not, you will be able to find someone you know easily. If we tested the whole population, a majority will have antibodies, and the mainstream medical world agrees with this.

If you do not have cold sores, or have never gotten one, all you have to do is the opposite of everything we've mentioned to promote good health. If it's healthy to rest, relax, avoid stress, avoid bad foods, and take nutrients, then it's just as easy to do the opposite to promote the opposite of health.

Be stressed. Don't sleep. Eat only junk food. Take drugs. Don't supplement – not even vitamin C! You will develop cold sores or something similar very quickly. You will get "sick", likely. You will likely develop growths all over the body in some form. Some of them could look like pimples, others like warts. You might even develop genital warts, whether you've ever had sexual contact or not. Cysts are likely. Rashes and fungal infections are likely. Respiratory infections are likely. Aches and pains and various discomforts will appear in short time.

I don't believe that you need to have sexual contact to develop symptoms of herpes, or the other H's. I believe all you need to do to show any of these symptoms is to be unhealthy. The more unhealthy, the more likely all the so-called H viral symptoms will appear.

And if you have symptoms, the whole list of things to do to promote health applies. The protocol from the allopaths is drugs that attack the immune system. We do not believe this is a good idea. There are many ways to support the immune system. I didn't mention extra zinc when talking about cancer, so I'll throw that in. It's another one of the essential nutrients that is also an antioxidant, and also supports and promotes a healthy immune system. It's also one of the few nutrients your doctor might actually say is a good idea to boost. If I had a diagnosis of an immune problem of any kind, including any virus, I would boost all of the antioxidant nutrients.

Many people survive a long time with HIV. I have an uncle who has had it as long as I have been alive. He's not in amazing shape, but he's alive. He looks like any other civilian on the street, in my opinion. Magic Johnson, once a posterboy of AIDS, is still alive. Magic Johnson for years has publicly endorsed various products that are said to "support the immune system."

Digging a bit deeper there are more sinister problems. The idea that many of the phony diseases came originally from animals, seems usually to be media nonsense. I'd recommend not listening to anything about health on TV. Even if you see me on TV, the edit is probably bogus. That wouldn't be a problem, except that humans tend to get the blame for the animal infection. In the case of AIDS, one man Gaëtan Dugas was publicly thought of as "Patient Zero." This vilification apparently harmed his life in a great way. I believe it.

We want to place blame on this *thing*, this noun. And if it is not a noun, a thing that can infect us, then this scam has hurt many people unnecessarily.

Certain groups were identified as being "more susceptible to AIDS." Let's have a closer look.

Gay men were singled out for two reasons. The first is anal sex. Rectal tissues are more easily damaged than vaginal tissues. The rectum does not secrete its own lubrication, but the vagina does. Anal sex is more likely to tare skin than vaginal sex.

Open wounds are susceptible to infections. Skin protects from infections. Both parties are liable to tare skin if inadequately lubricated, and this is a natural risk with anal sex. Obviously, the rectal cavity, if pierced, is at a high risk of infection.

That's one reason. They singled out gay men because gay men are more likely to practice anal sex. I think it's useful to teach safe practices for straight people too, by the way. But gay men were "at risk", so they were a lot of the focus.

The second reason they were singled out was because of party culture overlapping with gay male populations. They tended to party and do drugs. Especially amphetamine drugs that are known to be bad for the immune system. So they were also at high risk because of this. Drug users in general were also high risk, and gay men were known to overlap with that group quite a bit.

There's a few problems here. First of all, AIDS is a relatively new disease. Anal sex is not. It is as old as writing, as far as we know. Anal sex is inscribed on ancient tablets, and depicted in ancient statues and carvings. So there has always been a direct risk of infection present. The risk is not new.

Disinfection is also not new. There are a long list of plants and other antimicrobial things, like shell flour, essential oils, and fire, that the ancients knew about and most likely utilized to help deal with infections. They say the Incas were doing brain surgery, and I have to believe they knew about infections.

I have worked in one remote location, with no direct access to emergency medical care. It is a small village on the Pacific coast of Costa Rica. The entire Pacific Nicoya peninsula is known as a "blue zone", a place where people tend to live a long time, but that is another book. Most of the village does not speak English at all.

At my last count, two of the younger villagers were sent out to college. One of them learned massage therapy, a useful trade for the healthy tourist industry in the country, paid for with father's football money. The father now gets free massages and he already lives in one of the world's longest lived locations, and I think he's a pretty smart guy.

The jungle is known as a rough place for infections, and it's true. Fungus, bugs, birds, and all kinds of animals will steal your garden if you're not careful. Fungal infections in the body are likely if dampness is not kept in check. And spooky viruses are said to be ever present.

You might think that a people who have survived in an infection-prone environment for many generations would have many treatments for viruses. They don't. If you get hurt in the jungle, the remedy is usually sea water.

One of our students once stepped on a stingray. It punctured her foot. It was painful, but not threatening. She chose to stay in town, rather than venture the dirt roads many hours to a dodgy hospital.

Locals assured us that the hospital didn't have much for her anyway. She wasn't losing a lot of blood, and it was all wrapped up, but of course there is a risk of infection, which was our primary concern at that point. The local remedy: sea water. The foot stays in the sea water, it heals faster, it feels better, and it is less likely to get infected. Change the water frequently.

Once I had to crawl under a wooden deck to turn on a water main. I got many bullet ant stings. The local remedy was salt water.

Until 2015, I had only heard of one case of dengue fever in the area. Dengue is said to be a virus transmitted by mosquito. There are always a lot of mosquitoes in these hot damp places, which is part of the reason these places are known for many viruses. I do believe mosquitoes can make us sick.

That one case that I knew about was a student from a western country in a village down the road. She was not healthy generally, from what I was told. Her immune system was highly susceptible to infection, in my opinion.

But in 2015 something weird happened. A bunch of people got "dengue." They say in the tropics that dengue only gets you once, like chicken pox. Many people in the village had already experienced it at some point in their lives.

Dengue is miserable, like flu in paralysis. Wretchedly tired but unable to sleep. Sweating hot, freezing cold. The mandatory fan blowing on you to keep the mosquitoes away feels like little needles. This can last a few days or a week or more.

The worst part of the experience was *hydrophobia*. Very few other illnesses include hydrophobia, an intense repulsion to water. Rabies also has hydrophobia included in its symptoms. So dengue was like rabies with the flu, in paralysis. I'm just painting a picture here for you because we're talking about infections still. AIDS is still said to be an infection, but this is the kind of story I'm looking for when it comes to an infection.

So in 2015 nearly everyone in the village got what appeared to be dengue. They all called it dengue, because it felt like dengue to them. The village was getting quiet because everyone was at home in bed – you can't even pretend to go about your business with dengue.

We were getting pretty worried that we were going to get it too. Then there was a power outage that lasted longer than a normal rolling blackout. Long enough for the mosquitoes to really get us, without the fans on. Glass windows are a luxury in the jungle and so most people do not have them.

I remember it like it was yesterday. It was New Years Eve, and we were invited to a celebration at the Don's house. A Don is like an unofficial mayor. I was honored, frankly. But as we were getting ready, it hit me like a brick. I couldn't even really speak to my friends. I just crawled into bed and curled up, and stayed there for days.

My friends and I developed symptoms a few days apart, so we could help each other. We forced each other to eat, at least a little bit of egg or fish, and drink water and supplements. Saliva wasn't being produced, and chewing was very difficult. Like some chemical drugs, eating carbs or plant material is almost impossible. You can keep chewing and it doesn't seem to go anywhere. There is a real risk of choking.

We also forced each other to shower and go in the ocean. Actually we were already used to having our daily meetings in the ocean. We can get a short bit of vitamin D from the sun, a bit of a swim which is a nice luxury, and we can talk to each other without any distractions or devices. If I'm in charge of the time, I like to get extra value for the money.

With dengue, the beach and the water and the sun were all horrible. Painful even. If you can believe it, hydrophobia makes water disgusting. And we need water. Showering was miserable. Of course we didn't have hot water either.

One of my friends begged us to get him a helicopter airlift back to America or something. Anything, anywhere, anyone who could help. Many people begged God for it to stop or for a merciful death. I'm being dramatic because infections are dramatic, but honestly it was really horrible, and I prayed to God for it to stop too.

The local remedy, you can probably guess. Rest, try to nourish, salty water, and that's pretty much it. There is no shaman voodoo herb or root that will ease the suffering noticeably.

There were obvious differences in how people dealt with the problem. Everyone did a lot of resting as the primary treatment. But young people clearly got over it faster. None of us young people lasted longer than a week. Some old people lasted two.

Of the three of us, one was in great shape. He built himself a jungle gym and he forced himself to train weights and cardio during the dengue. I couldn't believe it even as I watched him. He looked like a zombie. It looked like torture, but he did it. And he forced the beach trip, which really was a five minute walk but seemed to take all day on dengue. He did it every day while myself and our other friend each took a couple days off.

Our fit friend got better faster than either of us. Much faster. His illness seemed really to only last 4 days. That was the village record.

Everyone called it dengue until the TV said that the rest of the world was saying there is something called Zika virus going around. So everyone switched to calling it Zika. It made sense to give it a different name anyway. It only felt like dengue, but we all understood dengue as a once in a lifetime deal. So it was probably something else.

I don't know exactly what a virus is, and I don't think anybody really does. But I do believe that we all caught something from a mosquito. Bugs can deliver pathogens into our bodies that attack us directly. I will tell another story in the next chapter, but suffice to say I am satisfied with labeling this phenomena a viral infection. It wasn't "terrain" that caused this, because we all got it, and the terrain didn't change. This is a healthier place than any other I have seen, and we all caught the infection.

The viral infections I'm familiar with mostly do not call for medicine, because few compounds have any reliable effect on the duration or outcome of viral infections. The duration and severity of the symptoms seem to depend on only two factors: the presence of the infection, and the state of the body dealing with it.

A less healthy body will be prone to more infections, and will have a harder, longer time dealing with them. Antiviral drugs suppress the immune system, that's what they say they do. I believe this further increases future potential of infections. An older body, or a body with an already existing digestive or immune issue or nutrient deficiency will deal with it less easily than a healthier person.

I am fine with calling a bug infection of any kind a "disease", even if the allopathic world doesn't have much to treat it, and neither do we. At least they could provide a safe and clean environment for you to wait out the infection. They could provide you with salt in an IV, one of the most useful things they do in my opinion. They could get you water and change your sheets and help you out. Grandma's method.

We could do that too but we're generally not equipped. Insurance doesn't pay us and neither do governments. So it's okay to go to a hospital if you have dengue, as long as you know that your chances are still about the same as they would be at home.

Does any of this sound like AIDS? We have a pretty good understanding about bacterial, fungal, and even viral infections when they are correlated to an infectious experience like Zika, or chicken pox. The way we diagnose AIDS is not by symptoms, like every other thing we have talked about until this chapter. The way we identify AIDS is to take a PCR test. It looks for markers, and depending on how many you have relative to the spectrum and the arbitrary distinction between HIV and AIDS, you are said to have one or the other. It doesn't matter what symptoms you have before you take the test.

The people who were identified for HIV tests were those at high risk of infection, and ill health generally. Those infectious risk categories included physical risk in the form of anal sex, and chronic risk in the form of drug users and "minorities." People who tend to be less healthy were identified as "at risk" for this "infection", and were given a test.

The groups of people they identified *are* at a higher risk of infections and chronic illness. These groups have lower life expectancy than others. People who use drugs do compromise their immune system. All drugs compromise the immune system. Fried food compromises the immune system. Cheap processed food compromises the immune system. Stress compromises the immune system.

All of this makes people more likely to get sick in many ways, specifically pathogenic illnesses. Cold, flu, sinus infections, yeast infections, ear infections, bladder infections. Regular sicknesses. This is the experience for unhealthy people, along with general aches and pains and headaches and so on.

If you look for particularly unhealthy groups, they're pretty easy to find. So we single those people out and say they are most likely to have these markers. And they're also likely to have other markers, such as HSV. They're also likely to get regular sicknesses regularly, and have many "antibodies" in the blood.

So we tell these people they have a disease. The treatment for the disease is antiviral or immune-suppressing drugs. If they survive for any length they are called an HIV or an AIDS patient. If they show improvement over arbitrary time, they can eventually be called "in remission." This is as far as the renaming can go. One is always a patient, whether they are in remission or not.

Many of the people who were told they had AIDS or HIV, or HSV for that matter, otherwise had no distinct symptoms. They had general symptoms. They had common health problems. My theory would be that the antiviral or immune-suppressing drugs didn't help any of these people get any healthier. Some of them publicly made lifestyle and nutritional changes and lived healthfully to a normal longevity. Many of them are still alive and I imagine they will continue to do well.

Some people didn't do the pharmaceutical drugs. Lots of people did. Many famous people died while on allopathic treatment programs for HIV or AIDS. It is usually said that these people died "*of* AIDS*"*, but this is definitely not clear. Dying of a heart attack is clear, but general immune failure is ambiguous as to the actual cause. Someone who dies of pneumonia should have pneumonia listed as their cause of death, not the presumed contributors to that immune failure. No death certificate should list AIDS as the cause of death, as that contributor to the final immune failure is speculative. Similarly, people who die of lung cancer should be said to have died from lung cancer, not smoking or obesity or any other presumed risk factor to the actual cause of death.

Even on the deathbed, the symptoms of AIDS are not unique to AIDS. The experience I described for dengue is quite unique. Syphilis is quite unique, with an easily identifiable pathogen. But AIDS patients tend to die of pneumonia. Pneumonia is essentially just final immune system failure. Kaput. It can happen to presidents if they stay out in the rain and catch a fever. I don't think the rain delivers a virus. I think the rain puts that last stress on an under-equipped system, and it fails.

The micro world is just waiting to devour us as soon as we stop breathing. A coconut drops from the tree and very soon after it is swarming with bugs and fungus and everything is moving in. I think it is the same in our bodies. If we let our internal environment tilt a bit, then bad bacteria, fungus, virus, and pathogens of all kinds are given the edge over us.

There is a word I have left out of the book so far: alkalinity. This is because there is so much hype behind the word that I like to distance myself from it. But let's cover it quickly.

Many people report success on helping people achieve a healthy immune system with natural methods. One such category is people with serious immune diagnoses, including AIDS. So, some people have claimed to get good results with AIDS patients, via lifestyle changes. If you believe any of the explanations in this book for the pathogenesis of disease, then this makes easy sense.

Some practitioners and patients attribute this success to the state of alkalinity. I have some technical disagreements, but as far as described here, I agree with the concept.

They say sugar feeds cancer, and sugar promotes acidity, the opposite of alkalinity. As far as I know, the most important factor for whether or not someone is alkaline, is whether they have enough calcium.

Calcium has many cofactors, and each is important, but none is more important for alkalinity. We have one cheap measure of alkalinity, and it's very reliable. Putting copper on the skin in the form of a bracelet or a wire will turn the skin underneath green, blue, or black, if the person is what we are calling "too acidic." If this happens, we say the person is not alkaline. There is a very small window of tolerance in blood PH. Too far in either direction is life-threatening very quickly.

I find the copper test very accurate. If I increase the stress on my day without increasing a spread of nutrients and water, then my skin will change color slightly. Most people will turn green quickly. But I will bet that any healthy person will show up green in a few hours if they ate a couple full sized bags of potato chips or a few candy bars. Calcium, water, and the water-soluble nutrients are the most important factors in reversing this quickly. Someone who is overweight might not lose the color under the copper until they have reached their proper healthy weight – this could take more than a year, but will happen if they continue to avoid the bad foods and take the adequate dose of the essential nutrients, particularly calcium and the others in the bone and joint group.

It is my opinion that the calcium product we promote is the best one in the world. It got me out of life long pain. And it keeps my skin clear while wearing copper. If I slack on it a few days, I will turn a bit green with my normal diet. Bone meal, wood ash, crop irrigation, and composting were the primary methods that "primitive" people used, without knowing the chemistry, to get more of these key minerals in their diets, and that lifestyle is simply unrealistic for those of us in the modern world.

Those water-soluble nutrients include all of the B vitamins, and vitamin C. Plants can make these things, and so we can get them in food and also in supplement form.

The water soluble nutrients include minerals called "electrolytes."

Sodium, potassium, chloride, calcium, magnesium and phosphorus are water soluble. Sodium chloride, salt, is water soluble and arguably the most important nutrient. Ancient soldiers are said to have been paid in salt at various times in history. This is where we get the word "salary." This is because you can pillage food all day, but you require salt to digest it. They couldn't cross deserts or mountains without it. Their animals couldn't either.

Salt has also been called the most alkalizing substance. Due to technicality, I have to agree. We need enough calcium to be alkaline, but we need salt to absorb calcium properly. We need salt for the stomach to work properly, and that function is important for all the rest of it. But salt on its own will not make you alkaline.

Using enough salt is required for having a healthy strong stomach acid, which is required for proper absorption of nutrients and digestion of food. If enough of all the essential nutrients are present, the person is alkaline and the body is not in a state of disease. Any person with any disease will likely experience the skin discoloration from copper. I would safely bet on it.

Since there is no identifiable link between a pathogen and the state of disease we call AIDS, and since there is no coherent "state of disease" for either AIDS or HIV, I can only assume this thing, sometimes referred to as an autoimmune disease and sometimes referred to as an infection, is neither. I believe the symptoms associated with HIV are symptoms of an unhealthy body, and the people claiming to help people achieve health by encouraging alkalinity, I believe them.

The hype about HIV/AIDS has decreased in recent years as new diseases come into fashion. But it is still big business, and it is still talked about today much the same way it was 30 years ago. Mainstream medicine still has no better odds with people now than they did when they first "discovered" it. In my business, since I can't "treat" diseases, I don't. I assume the person has an unhealthy immune system and I help them figure out how to support a healthy immune system.

The other H worth talking about before we move on is HPV. HPV is an even weirder case than AIDS, and totally deserving a good questioning. This is another H virus that is supposedly "caught" by skin to skin contact or sex.

Like HIV, HPV has no specific unique symptoms or experiences. People with HPV markers "may" develop warts or genital warts, and other common symptoms of a depressed immune system. If a woman with these symptoms is pregnant, she can give birth to a child with these symptoms also.

The CDC says 90% of HPV infections "go away on their own within 2 years." Very interesting. But you should still get a vaccine for it they say, of course. Never mind that the symptoms aren't that serious and will probably go away on their own without any treatment.

The weirdest thing about HPV in my opinion is the vaccine for it. The reasoning behind most of the marketing for this is that people with HPV markers are at a higher risk for certain cancers. But there is no vaccine that will "prevent cancer", and there is no vaccine that prevents infection from a fake disease. The symptoms of these H viruses are those of a generally unhealthy person, and a generally unhealthy person may indeed develop a form of cancer, because cancer is caused by the factors that make someone unhealthy.

If the H viruses were truly transmittable infections, a vaccine might make theoretical sense, except that vaccines do not *prevent* infection. A vaccine might make sense if it was sure to eliminate the risk of infection, but it does not.

To me it has not been properly demonstrated that any of the H's are infections. I think the blood can develop many antibodies as it is exposed to many things throughout life. The longer we live the more antibodies we may have. If we eat the wrong foods or are deprived of enough of the essential nutrients, we will face many challenges in life.

Some of those problems will be physical, mechanical problems. Others will be infectious. Some of those infections will be easily identifiable and treatable. Some will be pernicious, vague, and they can spell the end for the patient.

In any case, we know that none of the H's are a death sentence, and all of them have plenty of cases walking around just fine with no symptoms. I don't feel comfortable calling any of the H's a disease, or an infection, and I think this leads us perfectly into our final disease chapter, covering the latest fashionable disease.

10. The New Virus.

A few of the social media accounts I run could be considered "conspiracy" oriented. I am used to being on the outside opinion, but I am not used to much censorship about it. The only things that I was really directly censored about in the past were things that I considered fake news. Things shown on the news that I thought were fake, staged, directed, like a movie or a TV commercial. For whichever reasons, talking about fake news is discouraged on many social media platforms.

Since my accounts aren't about news, or fake news, this means I can usually say mostly whatever I want. All of the stuff in this book so far I am able to say on the internet or in public without expecting censorship. I have said everything here publicly before and posted it online.

In 2020 a new virus media event happened and suddenly I saw government links attached to my posts when my posts contained any word associated with the new virus. This now also happens to the word "vaccine."

I don't normally like to talk much about vaccines. I already know they are a target for censorship, and I really don't want my accounts punished in any way. We don't sell or promote anything having to do with vaccines, so it doesn't matter to the core of our message. There are books on the subject that I agree with, and I usually just recommend them and move on.[xxiv]

My point here is that these key words are in fact targeted for censorship. Since I am submitting this book to Amazon, I want to avoid these key words. So far this book is written in legal terminology that should not get me in trouble, but there are many new laws in place about this new virus that are much more worrisome than any disease we have so far discussed.

I will refer to this 2020 event as the "beer virus."[5]

At this point I want to say that I am not blaming any particular medical professionals for anything here. Bluntly, they are not educated in nutrition, and so I don't expect them to have a good understanding of most diseases we have covered. They also don't have to be bad people. I've worked in research and I know that all of us can have great intentions, yet the system can still be bad, and the outcomes can still be bad.

There might be more reprehensible deliberate obfuscations by the media, but even then I don't have the energy to assign personal blame. The media shouldn't be responsible for health information anyway, and neither should governments, in my opinion.

I believe there is a lot of deliberate misinformation, combined with a lot of good intentions gone wrong, combined with hysteria, combined with clumsy and controlled politicians who shouldn't be expected to know what to do about a pandemic. None of this would matter that much if it weren't for the consequences of closing down the world for nearly a year at the time of this writing.

Update: as of March 2022, the world has clearly changed dramatically in response to this pandemic. My home country of Canada has been nearly ruined economically, and I have shed tears driving through cities that used to thrive but are now boarded up. Like all the new laws that were put in place after the events of September 11, 2001, I do not expect any of the new government control systems put in place in response to the pandemic to ever be reversed. I have commented in more detail on the pandemic and the resulting "medical tyranny" in my book *Everything The Government Does Is*

---

5   Because of the popular beer "Corona."

Bad For Us.

I hope this sounds out of date to future readers and that everything did open back up and go back to normal, but I have a strong feeling that 2020 will be looked back upon as the year it all changed.

By the rest of this book it should be expected by my own logic that doctors should be responsible for handling this so-called pandemic. If it is an infection, which they say it is, and it has clear specific symptoms and experience, which they say it does, then it should be handled by professionals equipped to handle infectious disease.

But what if there is no disease?

I have gone to great lengths in this book to avoid using numbers, charts, studies, and unnecessarily technical language. Though the beer disease is arguably the most important event of our time, I still think we can make the argument for it being a fake without even using the exact numbers.

Though my training and experience is in nutrition, not medicine or infections, I do have some basic knowledge, and I know that if you look up "coronavirus" in a medical textbook, it will tell you that this type of virus is what we lay people call "the flu." Though there has been effort from the medical community to handle the flu pharmacologically, mostly through the use of annual flu shots, there has been little progress made in eradicating the flu. On a normal year, estimates tend to be in the range of 200,000-600,000 people killed worldwide from the flu.

These are estimates because exact cause of death in many cases, whether it is a presumed heart failure or some type of infection, are not often ascertained. Autopsies are rarely preformed, and different doctors and pathologists often disagree on exact cause of death. It is quite easy to declare with certainty that someone was killed by a bullet to the head, but is much more difficult with many of the common types of death, including the flu. So we will never have exact numbers on exactly how many people are killed by any virus, especially if they are already elderly or frail or have some other disease when they die of, say, a respiratory infection.

What we *do* know for sure is that this type of virus is not new, and neither are big numbers of people who die each year in association with different types of flu. The 2018-2019 season was a particularly bad year for flu cases worldwide, and yet there was no media-declared pandemic. Here I am not downplaying the seriousness of the flu or other common infections, especially pneumonia. These are serious threats that we need to be on top of. The best way to prevent any type of infection seems to be to *be healthy*. That statement sounds so simple that many people dismiss it outright, but all of the media outlets I have seen, as well as various government agencies in every country I have seen, have told us that the people most likely to die from this particular virus have at least two other existing health problems, especially diabetes, obesity, and some existing respiratory problem.

Further, although the mainstream world didn't talk much about it, many medical doctors and alternative practitioners heavily emphasized a few key nutrients and even herbs like pine needles in helping the body overcome such an illness. The most common nutrients that I saw touted were vitamin D and zinc, both of which are already essential nutrients, both of which are involved in numerous systems in the body which are no secret in nutritional science, and both of which can be legally claimed to "help support and promote a healthy immune system."

We are taught to *respond* to problems once they occur, and the primary way we do that in the modern world is to go to a doctor and consume some pharmaceutical compound. But pharmaceuticals in general have very low value when it comes to dealing with viruses. Bacteria are visible, because they have cells, and we can directly see whether a chemical agent – natural or pharmaceutical – kills the bacteria. This is not the case with viruses, and at best we have statistical associations to try to piece the truth together.

To us, "being healthy" means avoiding the bad foods, consuming all of the essential nutrients, and not much more. I do believe that exercise also helps a lot in staving off infections. I know some practitioners who recommend immediate vigorous exercise the moment you feel a sniffle or a tickle in the throat. We all know the feeling when we are "coming down" with something, and many people with a lot of experience believe that we can stop the sickness by refusing to "act sick." I don't have a way to quantify that belief scientifically, but it is definitely worth a try. I have already mentioned how our fit friend beat Zika faster than anyone else in our sample group, by doing exactly the same food and supplement regiment that we did, but adding vigorous exercise. I completely believe that his general fitness, combined with his food and nutrient habits, is what put him in a better position than any of us to beat the infection.

The media and governments across the world acted in 2020 like the flu didn't exist. Both the media and governments, to my knowledge, completely failed to acknowledge that the virus in question has always been listed as a flu virus. To my knowledge, the flu basically disappeared statistically in the years 2020 and 2021, because all such cases were recorded as cases of the beer virus. In my opinion, the flu did not disappear overnight, it was simply renamed. This statistical trickery is definitely not the only reason I consider this a fake disease.

As for this new pandemic with a not-at-all new virus, I would like to give you my opinion from the beginning. In late 2019 I was on the road. In Arizona, staying with a friend, the day before I was about to leave I did not feel good. I was "coming down with something", for sure.

I had been on the road for several months, and this was not the first sign that my body had had enough. I had been tired and hungry recently. My skin was showing blemishes and my lips were swollen. And now, for the first time in years, I was getting sick.

This was embarrassing because I am in the health business. I hadn't been sick like this since I started the program that I promote, and I knew *I* was to blame. Planes and cars are both heavy EMF, and can be generally exhausting. Staying with many different people all the time and shuffling from place to place is stressful. Eating can be a problem on the road, because I avoid common ingredients like gluten and oil, and so I also tend to eat very little while traveling. I also tend to drink more than my normal amount of coffee, which dehydrates, causing me to need more water-soluble nutrients like salt and vitamin C.

Normally I am not very hungry, but after a while on the road I can develop a serious craving. In America recently a few gluten-free cookie brands have also begun making "no oil" options. They're still not good. Sugar and processed carbs generally is still not good. But I was so hungry. I ate a bunch of them over probably a week and at the end of the week I got sick.

I'm confessing this for a few reasons. First, it shows that an other-wise healthy person can tilt that balance pretty easily. Second, it puts me in doubt that this viral experience I had was "caught." I don't think I got it from the cookies. I think I am more likely to get sick likely if I treat my body poorly.

This definitely was not a food-born illness. Anyone who has gotten a food poisoning knows that it is a very unique experience. There were none of the digestive symptoms in my sickness here. My pri-mary symptom was a miserable restlessness and lack of energy. Closer to dengue than to a bacterial infection.

The third reason to confess this is because this was Christmas Eve, and the latest disease being promoted was the beer virus. I had been using international airports and shaking hands and touching gas pumps, and I was at a high risk of picking up any bug with this lifestyle.

I spent Christmas day in a hotel in miserable restlessness. I spent as long as I could under the hot water in the shower. I drank lots of salty water and regular water. I doubled my supplements. I waited it out. I didn't eat anything because there is nothing good available at an airport hotel, especially on Christmas Day.

The next day I was well enough to travel to a friend's house and sit with her in miserable restlessness. After a few more groggy days, on New Year's Eve, I was just about normal and on the way back home.

Since we are in the health business, and our primary form of sales takes place in the form of answering questions from the public, we can expect questions about new diseases as they hit the news. Like vaccines, infectious diseases are not a topic I try to cover. We are not claiming to be emergency caregivers. We promote nutritional strategies for gradual and long term health improvements, mostly. We have to talk a lot about food and salt and other things, because it matters directly to our sales proposition. We are proposing that people will probably feel better and improve symptoms if they take our products, and we must insist that food matters in this equation.

The beer disease doesn't have anything to do with our business, and it is being targeted for censorship, so naturally I want to avoid the subject. But it kept coming up. People wanted to know what to do. We had the same answer to offer that we always do: support and promote the body's natural ability to maintain and repair itself. It was never very exciting, but people everywhere were excited about the beer virus.

I also think this answer was in line with what we can legally say. The news says there is a new flu out there, which is an immune problem. There are several things that are widely recognized as supporting and promoting a healthy immune system. Several of these indisputable compounds are also essential nutrients. Nutrients are deemed essential if we get a disease without them, but all essential nutrients will have multiple roles in the body, including the immune system.

Since the beginning of the new virus there was a flurry of activity around long known nutrients like zinc, vitamin C, vitamin E, vitamin D, and so on. These are essential nutrients and have always been a part of our pitch. So we didn't need to change this. Our recommendation remained the same: support the body by avoiding the bad stuff and taking all the essential nutrients in intelligent amounts. If attempting to further support the immune system, increase the specific nutrients that are known to do this. They are called antioxidant nutrients. Increasing all the water-soluble nutrients is not a bad idea either.

A lot of people expected us to jump on this pandemic as a way to market these specific nutrients more heavily. But we have never recommended just taking one or a few nutrients. We have always recommended taking all of them and boosting some as needed.

I didn't change my habits in response to the growing concern. I didn't buy hand sanitizer. I only use hand sanitizer if we are out in the forest without running water. Otherwise I wash my hands with soap and water and that's all.

Early in 2020 we were in Michigan with my mentor, Dr. Joel Wallach. He's a veterinarian, a comparative pathologist, and a naturopathic human physician. I figure he knows more about these beer viruses than I do. Every time I see him I try to have a few questions. As the years have gone on, I have had less questions. I think this is because I believe myself to understand most of the topics that come up. This is good.

But in the nutrition business we are not supposed to be experts on viruses. Surgeries and infections can be very complicated. It's something people go to school for. It's professional territory requiring licenses and qualifications that I don't have. Dr. Wallach has those credentials, so I asked him.

He gave me the same answer that he gave the audience that evening. He said that beer viruses are common. They are a type of flu. The flu kills many people each year. Some years they have different names, but it's more or less the same thing. At this time the talk on the TV was mostly still about China and Europe.

The TV and others said that this beer is different from the beers of history. This one is especially potent, they say. In the early months I saw a lot of footage of people in China falling over in the street from this "virus." I am not familiar with any virus that strikes a person so violently.

There were also many people laying down apparently dead in the street. It looked apocalyptic. And it looked very strange. I have seen at least one virus hit an entire small population hard, as described in the AIDS chapter. Everyone went to bed. They did not go out on the streets to lay down on a staircase. What we were seeing in China was very strange.

This type of behavior could have been caused by two things, in my opinion. The first is some sort of radiation stun. Crowd control. There are frequency-based stun technologies. I assume these could be made strong enough to kill a person, but from the footage I have seen it is not clear if any of the people laying down were dead. Many of them break their own fall as they are falling, which looks like acting. And many move while on the ground. There are lots of videos showing this.

I know these are very strong claims and so I made a full length video about it. The video was taken down from YouTube and blocked from Bitchute. I managed to get one version of it onto my Instagram account @TranscendTowers, but then I decided to make an extended version and put it on its own website. It is probably worth writing a book on the subject, but it was well suited to a video.

The video can be viewed on www.WagTheDogTheory.com. I recommend downloading it if it is still up when you check. I could have included hours of the people falling down, but there is much more relevant content to make the case in the video.

On the video I attempted to establish that the media has a history of participating in, or falling for fake news stories. In the 1997 movie Wag The Dog, the main characters in the film stage a short clip about a war with Albania, to avoid a sex scandal with the president. It is an entertaining and instructive watch. I believe this concept has given us many incidents to talk about, including the 2020 event.

My strongest reason for saying this, apart from the many strange things in western media, is this Chinese falling down dead phenomenon. It appears as if these people were either being stunned, or that some or all of them were acting. This behavior was not seen anywhere else in the world. If they had a virus that was dropping people like that, why did it not look like that anywhere else? Was it a different virus? Was it a virus at all?

My wife suggested that I remove these paragraphs from the book. She said the rest of the book doesn't sound like a conspiracy, but this does. She has seen our platforms punished for talking about the beer virus in general, and she knows that I have very little to gain by covering this topic, as it is indeed a conspiracy theory.

She is right. The point of this book has nothing to do with this pandemic. And the pandemic has nothing to do with our business. We help people understand and overcome common chronic problems. We don't do pandemics, it's not in our job description or training. But the pandemic has changed our world, affected my own life and the lives of people that I love, and I care quite a lot about that.

I am compelled to offer some kind of theory to explain the people falling down in China. There has been very little commentary offered about it from either the mainstream or the alternative world. It seems most people forgot about this happening, or they never saw the footage. It was only shown briefly, before the script moved on. I saved hours of this footage and I have watched it deeply and it still does not make sense.

There has not been any other virus promoted using this type of footage that I am aware of. I have lived through many viral scares so far, including SARS, bird flu, Ebola, Zika, mad cow disease, etc. I cannot recall ever seeing footage of anyone falling down from any virus, anywhere in the world. Hollywood movies really don't even look like that. When hit with a virus, people tend to slow down dramatically, but they don't just drop dead on the streets. That's what weapons do.

Since there is nothing to compare the footage to, I have to come up with something. And since no one that I am aware of has really talked deeply about this footage, I don't have any other theories to reference. Lots of people blamed this phenomenon on 5G cell phone towers being "turned on." I thought I was being reasonable to assume this was not the case – especially as, again, the falling down phenomenon hasn't to date happened anywhere else, yet 5G is supposedly "on" all over the world.

In the footage, there are only select people falling over. It is not whole crowds. It does not look to me like a tranquilizer, and there is no evidence of that as far as I can tell. It also does not look like poisoning. There are no bodily fluids – blood, pus, urine, foaming at the mouth, nothing – or other signs of poisoning. There is also no clear evidence that any of the people falling over or laying down are dead.

There is clear evidence in most of the videos that most of the people on the ground are moving by themselves, so they are alive. There is also footage of people in body bags moving, and opening their eyes. These, to me, are clear proof of staging a media event, not the recorded documentation of actual people dying. Again these claims required video evidence to prove, which is why I made the video. In most of the footage, none of these people are coughing or communicating at all. They could be stunned or they could be acting and I honestly have no other theories. Maybe they were drugged, but it just doesn't look like that.

This is important evidence that was used to implement the most serious "disease" protocol ever seen on Earth by anyone alive. Then
this evidence disappeared from all conversation except the hard-
core conspiracy theorists who still say 5G must be responsible.

I would be fine calling the beer virus the thing responsible for the
people falling down. But I would have questions about the rest of
the world. China seems to be doing fine at the moment, without
people falling down in the streets. People didn't fall down anywhere else, no matter their ethnicity or country of origin.

Videos are better than numbers in some cases. But the numbers for
the beer disease have been questionable from the start. Deaths by
chronic diseases like heart attack and cancer nearly disappeared
during the pandemic, as did the regular flu that tends to kill around
250,000-500,000 people a year according to the World Health Or-
ganization. The numbers are further complicated by the difference
between dying *with* and dying *from* a disease, and this distinction
has been a problem through the whole pandemic – again, the
mainstream has told us that the people who are dying by and large
have more than 2 existing health problems.

In other words, the people most likely to die are already unhealthy.
An unhealthy person who dies "with" an infectious agent present
probably did die *from* that infection, and I argued in the previous
chapter that the ultimate cause of death *should* be what appears on
the death certificate, not any presumed "risk factors" that may have
contributed to their overall susceptibility. Nonetheless, there are
many important questions and distinctions that have really been
left out of the conversation. To understand disease and susceptibility to disease, we do need to clarify these very important concepts,
such as the fact that if you are unhealthy, you are more likely to die
from an infection. This is important because we are told that if we
look at the entire population, we citizens as a whole have less than
a 1% chance of dying from this particular infection, which is about
the same chance of dying if you contracted the flu on any year of
your life.

All of us were affected by the lockdowns, mandates, and economic
and emotional hardships caused by the response to this virus, and
yet there was a well-known elevated risk only for unhealthy and el-

derly people. Children have almost no chance of dying from this virus, and yet they were forced to cover their faces and distance themselves from other humans during their most critical years for social and psychological development. I feel a deep sorrow for any children who had to experience these unwarranted protective measures. Here I am not even making the case that the virus itself is fake, I am making the case that it was never reasonable to respond to the flu in this way. It would have been reasonable to focus attention on the groups – unhealthy and elderly – who were most at risk, but I would still not support removing rights from anyone or closing businesses in response to the threat level even for those most at risk. The risk was not high enough, even for the at risk people, and I believe in freedom strongly enough that I believe at risk adults should remain free to make their own choices regarding voluntary segregation or covering their faces and so on.

Several people have speculated that this virus was manufactured in a lab in China. Even if this were the case, the apparent risk of this new virus was no greater than the common flu viruses. Even with possible inflated numbers – people who actually died from something else but were recorded as a death from the beer virus – there was no excess mortality in the years 2020 or 2021. The world population *increased* during this time, as it has every year for well over a century. Even if it were a particularly deadly flu, it isn't significantly more problematic than many other years in living memory, such as the 2018-2019 season.

To me, all of these numbers and factors still distract us from my main reason for calling this pandemic an orchestrated media event: the clearly fake footage of people dropping dead in China. There is no explanation for the people falling down other than some kind of manipulation. Those people were either dropped with some kind of weapon, or they were acting, and in any case no government or media outlet has bothered to try to explain it. Again, these people falling down were the initial reason for the very serious response in other countries, and everything that followed stemmed from that. If the initial reason for the lockdowns and mandates were faked, then the pandemic itself is a fake event, created by media and politicians for reasons we can only speculate about.

We are used to seeing the types of symptoms that have been reported in the west. Flu-like symptoms. Respiratory infection type symptoms. We alternative people don't have ventilators to offer, and quite honestly I didn't even understand the use of one before they were in the news. At the beginning of the event I misspoke on podcast, calling them respirators. We don't use them, so I didn't know. But I didn't see how they could be helpful.

The story behind the ventilators, is that the human body doesn't like having a tube jammed down the throat. We tend to have to give serious drugs to a person, to get them into a state where they can receive such "treatment." One of these drugs is fentanyl, which by mainstream accounts, kills many people on its own. I consider deaths from fentanyl to be a pandemic in itself, especially from street drugs being "laced" with it. Several people that I know, all of them under the age of 40, have died in recent years from fentanyl "overdose." In the small town I live in, Kirkland Lake, Ontario, fentanyl appears to be the leading cause of death.

I am told by people who do know about ventilators that in some cases they can truly save someone's life. I am sure there are some emergencies where they are warranted, but the mainstream media reported that upwards of EIGHTY PERCENT of people who were put on ventilators during the pandemic, died. 80% is much more than the less than 1% risk of dying from the virus itself – would you rather face an 80% chance of dying, or a more than 99% chance of surviving without treatment? To me, an 80% death rate from this "treatment" is mass murder. I assume that if ventilators were not part of the response to this virus, many more people would have survived, which would have put the actual percentage of people at risk of dying even lower than the already-low figure of less than 1%.

My own grandfather recently died on a ventilator. He didn't have the beer virus. He called my mother from the hospital, telling her that he was basically fine and would be home the following day. That evening, for some reason, the hospital decided to put him on a ventilator, and he was dead soon after. I assume it is the drugs they put him on before even putting the tube in that really killed him, and I assume many other people were submitted to these drugs and the tube down the throat completely unnecessarily. He was old and in my opinion he should not have been put on any drugs, because his age and existing health conditions put him at a high risk of dying from such drugs. Fentanyl kills plenty of young people who do not have diseases, and it is much more likely to kill an older person with other health problems.

Why someone with an infection would want to go through this is beyond me, but I assume that most of them didn't even have a choice. And of course, these people had been bombarded with propaganda about a "deadly" virus for several months, and have been culturally conditioned to "trust the doctors." If the real risks of death were presented honestly, and people were given a choice about the ventilators based on reasonably "informed consent", I assume many would have chosen to just go home rather than face a near certain death on a ventilator. Even worse is the fact that most of these people were deprived of the ability to see their loved ones one last time, again under the false pretenses of a "deadly viral threat."

I would rather go to a sauna than a hospital. The numbers they report as success with the ventilators are terrible. This treatment, in response to this virus, is definitely not a success. On my end of the Q&A world, every person who has reported to me that someone died of the beer disease, said they were on a ventilator. All of them. In the two years we have been dealing with this pandemic, I have not yet had one person tell me of anyone they know who died without being on a ventilator. This is not a quantified fact, it is only based on reports I receive, but you would think that at least one person would have told me that someone they know actually died of this thing at home or in any other situation than on a ventilator.

Many people reported that they were tested positive, or they developed something like the news was describing, a respiratory flu. They got better. No one who died, reported to me, did so at home. They were all on a ventilator. I repeat this to emphasize my conclusion that most of the deaths that were reported as victims of the beer virus, were actually victims of murder from a horrendous treatment procedure. But this was really the main treatment offered by the allopathic profession. It seems more than sloppy to me. There were even a few pharmaceuticals that had reported success against the virus, yet this information was severely suppressed and censored on both mainstream media outlets, and social media. Regular medical doctors and alternative practitioners and researchers had their posts deleted, or their accounts disabled or deleted, because they talked about *successful* pharmaceutical treatments that did not include a ventilator. I guess they really wanted us on ventilators.

There are some pharmaceuticals that I believe are very helpful. They can save lives, definitely. Short-term use of some pharmaceuticals is included in the necessary toolkit we humans have at our disposal, particularly for acute problems like infections and accidents. If you get hit by a car, I have no problem with you taking pharmaceutical painkillers. Vitamins and minerals will not help you as much in the immediate term. Vitamins and minerals are required for *long-term* health and longevity, not for dealing with the immediate consequences of accidents or infections. This simply does not apply to chronic problems like most of what we have covered in this book – long term pharmaceutical use is unanimously bad.

Having said all of that, if certain pharmaceuticals *did* show a better result than the awful results of ventilators, I would be all for it. If they save lives, use them, short term. I thought that most of the censorship on social media and regular media was about *natural* things like zinc and vitamin D, or herbal concoctions. I thought these outlets were "in the pocket" of pharmaceutical companies, and wouldn't censor a positive outcome of a pharmaceutical drug. I was wrong, and it seems to me that the real interest of these companies is to promote the use of ventilators. This conclusion troubles me deeply, because it suggests that *despite* the obvious allegance to pharmaceutical companies, media outlets would rather see us dead on a ventilator than use a pharmaceutical drug.

Even as numbers rose on the television for the two years of the pandemic, I haven't in this whole time seen or heard of anything that looks like something other than a flu. I haven't seen or heard of anything like Chinese people falling over in the streets. Chinese people in western cities did not fall down in the streets. Many people have gotten sick. Many people get sick every year. If the period we are measuring is now over a year, the chances are very good that many people would have been sick of something like this in this time frame.

I don't know what the beer virus really is. From what I can tell, there is a flu present. Maybe 2020 was a worse year than normal, like 2018, a relatively bad year for flu viruses. I can't tell if it was a bad year because the numbers don't make sense. Other deaths from chronic diseases don't just disappear, and neither does the regular flu if there's a new one that year.

I also don't trust PCR tests and I never did. The guy who invented them said you could use the test to find whatever you want. I believe him.

What I do know is that I have never experienced this type of totalitarianism in response to a "health crisis." I am tempted to pause for a tirade about my personal inconveniences during the closures and lockdowns, but I have complained loudly elsewhere. My life has been interfered with in ways I have never experienced from governments before. I have never seen economies forced to halt.

The legal entitlement of a disease falls under the jurisdiction of licensed medical professionals. One consequence of this entitlement is that this profession is licensed to deliver medicines and other treatments in response to disease. The 2020 event is called a disease, therefore, this is the jurisdiction of the medical profession.

Though I have many problems with the classification of disease, I do not have a problem with this legal entitlement, when appropriate. One benefit of licensing the care of practitioners, is that politicians cannot legally deliver medicine or give medical advice.

My primary contention with chemical fluoride added to public water supplies is *not* that it is harmful. It could be beneficial, I don't care. It requires proof to demonstrate an effect either way, and I don't want to deal with proof. We can handle such questions with logic.

Fluoride is added in the water not for purification purposes. Chlorine is added to water for purification purposes. I have a separate problem with that, for another day. Fluoride is added into public water supplies for a medical purpose. The medical purpose is to prevent tooth decay. That's the reason they give for adding the stuff. But since this is a medical purpose, by law, this is the jurisdiction of medical professionals. This is a medicine, to treat a health problem – tooth decay. Doctors are supposed to be the only profession licensed to prescribe medication for health problems.

People, in this system, are supposed to retain the choice of which medicines to put in their body. They are supposed to be informed on the known benefits and risks of the proposed treatment. They are supposed to give their "informed consent" to the treatment, *after* discussing the benefits and risks. Ultimately, what they do in response to a medical problem is their choice – their doctor works for them, they do not have to take the doctor's advice. They don't have to fulfill the prescription or go on a ventilator, or cover their face and so on. Politicians are not doctors and should not be allowed to prescribe medication to anyone, let alone entire populations.

In my profession, I'm expected to give some kind of disclaimer that my advice is not legally acceptable medical advice. And I expect media and politicians to adhere to the same guidelines.

My problem with fluoride is political. I don't care if doctors think it will help my teeth or not. I don't feel the need to use it, and I care about my choice to make that decision. Doctors are there as an option. I can go and see my doctor, and ask his advice. I can choose whether to take his advice or not.

My problem with the new disease is also political. I don't really care what viruses are floating around this year or next. I am prepared to face the world to the best of my ability. I choose to support my body's ability to deal with infections, by supporting my immune system. I would like to use dramatic words to express my disappointment in my home country, Canada, essentially devastating its own way of life. But to be brief, I don't think business as usual will continue anytime soon. I think unreasonable measures against an invisible threat will continue and may increase. I think this fake event has been used to implement new rules, laws, and government agencies whose sole purpose is to reduce our personal power, freedoms, and legal rights, while tightening the overall control of our lives. I want to hope that borders re-open and that sanity restores, but I am not willing to bet on it.

Update: the border between the US and Canada has officially re-opened, technically. But I have been denied four times now trying to cross with my car. I am married to a US citizen, and my residence application is in process. I have crossed the border numerous times over many years, and I have always returned when I said I would. I have no criminal record in either country, and no current criminal charges. I have been denied entry a total of six times over the years, (including the four times during the pandemic), but my record is one of compliance. I was denied for things that I was honest about, not for smuggling or any form of dishonesty.[xxv] Though the border is technically open now, and despite my record of compliance, I was still denied entry recently at the supposedly "open" border. They told me to turn around and fly into America. I wasn't being denied entry entirely, I just was not allowed to cross with my car.

Of course, if the goal is to reduce contact between people to reduce the risk of spreading infection, then telling me to fly instead of drive makes absolutely no sense – I will be in contact with far fewer people on the road than in airports and planes. So I do not consider the border to be "open", particularly as both countries now require proof of vaccination to enter. This extortion has removed the right for a citizen of either country to exercise informed consent, and is not representative of a "free" country, or an "open" border.

There will always be pathogens around. We will always need to support and promote a healthy body and immune system. Chances are, we will still get sick a few times in life. None of this is new. But the world has changed dramatically because of what I believe to be a fake disease. And my biggest concerns about it are all political.

Doctors don't even seem to have much to do with this mess. The frustration felt by the people and the draconian measures imposed are from politicians, not doctors. As far as I can tell, the people behind this pandemic are media spokespeople and politicians. Even Dr. Anthony Fauci, has not been an actual medical practitioner for decades. He doesn't see patients, he works with the government on political responses to health issues. He is a researcher and a politician, in my opinion, and despite knowing everything we have covered in this chapter, he chose to promote medical tyranny instead of a reasonable medical response.

Incidentally, Dr. Fauci was also the main figure behind promoting the AIDS scare decades ago, and in the opinion of many, including myself, he is largely responsible for everyone who died taking the drug AZT rather than supporting their immune systems. AIDS was the first time that the PCR test was used to diagnose a "disease", and inflame public fear about a disease, and back then Kary Mullis, the guy who invented the PCR test and got the Nobel Prize for it, called Fauci a liar and worse, challenged him to debate, and denounced the use of the test for diagnosing the disease. It does indeed seem that Fauci has no interest in honestly communicating what he knows about diseases. This tendency towards dishonesty and sensationalism, I guess makes him a typical politician.

None of what has happened in response to this virus should've happened, because these are medically based decisions, and it was never the business of politicians to make medical decisions for us. We always should have had the choice of whether to use fluoride or not, or subject ourselves to experimental medications or not, or cover our faces or quarantine ourselves, etc. Informed consent no longer exists in the world of medical dictatorships we now live in.

That is the best I can do on this subject without detailed analysis. If this is a real virus, I think the response to it is much worse than the infection. Others have said that the cure should not be worse than the disease, and I completely agree.

11. What is Disease, Really?

Many years ago I arrived late one night at my friend's apartment. He wasn't there but he knew I was coming. I had been staying there throughout the summer.

We had badly neglected the lawn that summer. The grass was long and full of bugs and other creatures. The door was locked but the basement window in the back was not locked.

I crawled into the house and I brought fleas in with me from the long grass outside. I know this happened because I had just been there, and there were no fleas. I was tired and I slept on the couch with my clothes on. And I woke up covered in fleas.

I also woke up in another mental dimension. Something was amazingly wrong. Psychedelically wrong. Everything was wrong. I didn't know where or who I was for a moment. The room was kaleidoscopic and I did not feel good at all.

I made it to the bathroom. The ten foot distance felt like it took a while, but I didn't trust my perception of time. I felt drunk but also very sick. In the mirror, I was as pale as ever and I was bleeding from my nose. My eyes were bloody red as well.

I used the toilet and there was a lot of blood. None of this had ever happened to me before. I was delirious and it felt hard to even think about what was going on.

I called my mother. She is a school teacher and she happened to work right across the street from my friend's house. I told her I needed her help, and I dragged myself over to her office.

I had a feeling that I didn't need to go to the hospital. I figured I needed antibiotics, and fast. She took me to our family doctor. He agreed with my prognosis, wrote up a prescription for antibiotics, and I picked them up at the pharmacy downstairs.

I took the drugs, and I began to feel better quite quickly. I really was worried for a moment. I had never been bleeding from everywhere before. I felt like I was going to die, and I believe to this day that conventional medical treatment saved my life that day.

I stayed with my mother for a few weeks. In that time, I rested a lot. I watched a lot of TV on the couch with blankets and hot beverages and soups, and that's pretty much it. Modern grandma's recipe.

I don't have anything personal against my doctor. There is a certain hostility that can be found in the alternative world for the failures of the modern medical professions. A certain indignation. Righteous indignation. Many people who have found alternative paths to health carry an underlying outrage that their conventional doctors failed to help them.

I was born with health problems and I grew up with pains in many forms. My doctor could have known about the nutritional strategies that eventually did get me out of pain. When I did eventually find the right doses of the right stuff I needed, the pain I had been living with for 25 years disappeared in less than a week.

I am, deep down, upset that I missed so many healthful years. I could have thrived in my youth, but I was held back by chronic pain. It is unfortunate that my doctor, and his profession, is not required to learn about nutrition, because it was nutrition that eliminated my symptoms. But it's not his fault. It's a shame.

My mother also didn't know that her nutrition would cause problems in me. Also not her fault, also unfortunate. And it is unfortunate that my pain, and most of the pain we deal with in the public, was preventable and reversible long ago.

When I caught that bug from that flea, it was pretty clear what had happened. When I tell the story, I don't refer to the incident as a disease. I caught a particularly horrible bug.

My doctors gave me a few potential disease names for the pains and problems I experienced growing up. The names never seemed to matter, because the explanations were vague and unsatisfying, and the treatments offered were usually harmful. I didn't like pharmaceutical drugs and they didn't seem to help my pains anyway.

I got better results with over the counter pain creams than from decades of searching for answers from my regular doctor. And then I was completely relieved of the main problems that had bothered me a lifetime, in under a week. Hopefully having said all of this, you can see my point of view about the nature of disease.

So, what is a disease?

Aside from the legal aspect of the word, a disease is a belief. In some cases, such as syphilis, we can easily identify a pathogenic cause. It is sensible to believe in bugs, because they can get us, and we need to act when that happens.

But everything else we have talked about is a name for a cluster of symptoms. Symptoms are all the result of unhealthy bodies. Various things can contribute to stresses, and various things can defend against them. It doesn't seem useful to think of these things as diseases.

Sometimes we are presented with a new disease, and I think we ought to ask serious questions about these new diseases. I think we should retain the legal rights to support our body the way we choose, and take the medical advice we choose. I do not think governments should be empowered to make health decisions for individuals, or groups.

For the common health challenges that face so many people in my country and others, I encourage a shift in the way we think about disease. Identifying as a diseased patient, or "having" a disease that is not transmitted, is not correct or helpful.

Thinking about most diseases as something we "catch" rather than something we encourage or discourage, does not help us understand the nature, development, prevention, or reversal of the symptoms. It does not lead us to better treatment. It leads us further into the mess of the medical establishment.

No one should be on long term medication for health problems that are preventable, or reversible. And none of us should fear diseases that don't exist.

I think we should stop using the word "disease." If we catch an infection, we can simply refer to it as an infection, and we should all be able to understand what is happening. If our body is failing us or falling apart, there is no practical value in calling this process a disease.

Dis-ease, "a lack of ease, once-well but not now", this might have been what the word once meant. Now it means anything the medical industry wants research and treatment money for. Dis-ease isn't cured with medical treatment, and it never will be.

The medical world now wants to call practically everything a disease. They want to "treat" obesity and depression under the same legal umbrella as infections and accidents. When something is called a disease it can be paid for by insurance. Whether the treatment works or not is not the business of the insurance companies – they trust the medical establishment to define disease and treatment appropriately. The medical establishment has failed us deeply by giving a disease name to everything from anxiety to addiction.

The absolute best that medical treatment can do, is ease or relieve symptoms, often at the cost of another function in the body. The medical industry has a terrible track record even for this. The mainstream medical industry cannot currently cure heartburn, yet we trust them with cancer. Our alternative industry only exists because so many people fail to find relief from the mainstream professions.

We do not need to put common health problems and degeneration in the care of licensed professionals. We can take care of ourselves and live a long healthful life.

I and others are committed to helping average people understand the root causes of their health problems, and offer them advice on how to reverse those problems. If you found this book helpful, I ask that you share it with someone you know. Together we can create a healthier world, and it starts with this information. I for one do not want to see any of my friends or family complain about common aches, pains, weight problems, headaches, and the many minor symptoms the average person accepts as "normal", and I definitely don't want any of them to struggle with a chronic problem that their doctors would call a disease.

If you would like specific advice from us regarding yourself or someone you know, I encourage you to contact us. Our contact information is in the *More* section of this book. We promise to respond to every message, and to give you our best advice, for free, as long as we live.

The same principles that relieve minor symptoms also apply to more serious issues. People tend to get freaked out by scary words like "cancer", and "autoimmunity", but the nutritional advice for supporting the body's ability to be healthy and heal itself is the same for headaches as it is for miscarriages and diseases named after German doctors that you've probably never heard of.

If a doctor tells you that a disease is genetic, you can take that to mean that they have no idea what causes, prevents, or reverses that problem. Blaming genes is only the latest scapegoat in a long history of failed disease theories. Your great grandmother might have been told that "bad humors" were the cause of her health problems, and that is as true as the current genetic theory of disease transmission.

Genes are dependent on the environment, and though I avoided technical discussion in this book, you should know that it is now approaching conventional wisdom that this is true. We know that genes have not changed much in the last hundred years, but the prevalence of diseases have changed dramatically. Our environment — food, EMF, stress, nutrient availability — has changed, not our genes. We can rectify most of the problems caused by the modern way of life, by eliminating the worst of the foods in our grocery stores, and adding the nutrients that are missing from the food.

If it hasn't been made clear already, pharmaceutical drugs are not the answer to chronic disease. Your doctor will not tell you that the blood pressure drug will "cure" your blood pressure problem. At best, it will "manage" the problem, and if the doctor is honest they will tell you that the list of expected side effects are much longer than the one potential benefit of reducing the blood pressure. The same is true for all drugs that are marketed to manage symptoms – none of them deal in any way with the root problem, and none of them are expected to permanently reverse the symptoms. The only way to permanently reverse symptoms is to permanently change the factors that caused the symptoms, and unfortunately this is something doctors are not required to know anything about.

If you are shot with a bullet, hit by a car, or show symptoms of a serious infection, you should go to a medical doctor. Everything else is in your control.

Epilogue

After this book was first published I realized that I had missed one very common and very fake disease that comes up all the time in our daily dealings with the public: sleep apnea. Sleep apnea isn't a disease, and actually isn't even a problem. Sleep apnea – the temporary cessation of breathing while sleeping – is a completely normal behavior in all mammals. All mammals periodically stop breathing when they are asleep. This is yet another thing that has been declared a disease simply because human researchers and practitioners are not educated on animal nutrition or behavior.

Probably because sleep researchers only study sleep, no one seems to have noticed that people – and animals – also periodically stop breathing *during the day*. Unless you pay attention to it, you probably don't take full breaths either. Most people, most of the time, only expel half of the air in their lungs, leaving the bottom half stagnant and unrecycled. This is why "conscious breathing" is something we recommend all the time, and all it means is to pay attention to your breathing, and take full deep breaths more often.

Deep breathing has an immediate relaxing effect. When we are in "fight or flight" mode we breathe more rapidly and less fully. Our world isn't exactly set up to help us relax, and one of the consequences of a stress-filled life is the lack of full deep breaths. Several meditation techniques focus *only* on the breath, and everyone who has reported improvements with such programs is proof of how important breathing is.

Nobody needs a machine to help them sleep. People do report improvement with the CPAP (continuous positive airway pressure) machines, but that "treatment" is missing the cause of the problem. Apnea is not the problem, because apnea is normal. People go to sleep clinics because they have *other* sleep problems. Snoring, restlessness, and breathing problems in general have nothing to do with apnea. Snoring and breathing problems are probably caused by a digestive problem – which prevents key essential nutrients from being absorbed, which are responsible for lung function. Lung problems are nutrient problems, and possibly bacterial problems. These are food and nutrient problems, again having nothing to do with the temporary cessation of breathing that we call apnea.

Being overweight is the most common "risk factor" for having one of these sleep problems. Being overweight is bad for the body in general. A body isn't functioning optimally if it is overweight. If the body is lacking in the nutrients we need for proper lung function, the person might have a sleep problem. These people will *also have problems during the day.*

Insomnia itself is a mineral deficiency – the bone & joint group of minerals govern muscle function, and insomnia is a muscle problem. When you go to a sleep clinic with insomnia, they may very well just say that you have "sleep apnea" as an overall attempted explanation. The CPAP machine might help the person sleep better, but in my experience if they don't deal with the food problems and nutritional deficiencies, they will still have trouble sleeping.

You don't have to be overweight to have a sleep problem or a breathing problem, but it happens more in overweight people than otherwise. Malabsorption or outright deficiency in the "good fat" nutrient group can cause breathing problems in skinny people too. It can also cause people to be unable to *gain* weight. The point here is that the diagnosis of apnea does absolutely nothing to address any of these problems. People with sleep problems or breathing problems need to get off the bad foods and consume all 90 essential nutrients, appropriate to their body weight.

I also realize that I didn't really mention heart disease, the most common cause of death in the world. The first thing to note is that *something* will kill all of us. If we live to 120, it will probably be a heart attack or stroke that finally kills us, and likely on a cold night, in our sleep. This means that you can die peacefully of "age", and still be listed as a "victim" of heart disease.

There are several types of heart disease, and all of them are nutritional. Again, eventually the heart will fail, even if we are totally healthy, but many people die *prematurely* of a heart failure in some form. The bad foods contribute to heart problems in at least two ways. First, problematic grains impede the absorption of the fatty nutrients most prominently, and several of these nutrients are directly involved in heart health. Look at the label of any omega 3 product on the shelf and it probably says "may prevent heart attack and stroke." The reason they are able to say this on the label is because this is a "qualified health claim" granted by the FDA – after Dr. Joel Wallach sued them over it.

A qualified health claim means that sufficient evidence has been presented to legally make this claim. Before Dr. Wallach sued the FDA over omega 3 *supplements*, it was already legal to claim that "eating foods rich in omega 3 may prevent heart attack and stroke." More simply, it is well-established that this one nutrient deficiency is a factor in heart attack and stroke. The claim extends to various forms of thrombosis as well, because thrombotic problems are essentially a problem with blood clotting, and the fatty nutrients, particularly omega 3, are required for the blood to maintain proper viscosity. Blood is supposed to clot at certain times, but in a state of fatty nutrient deficiency it is liable to clot inappropriately, causing a clog in the artery, potentially leading to a heart attack or stroke.

Cardiomyopathy heart attack, (also called enlarged heart, athlete's heart, and sometimes "a genetic heart condition"), is linked to another extremely important nutrient, selenium. Selenium is fat-soluble and thus is part of the "good fat" group that comes up again and again when talking about common diseases. Selenium and omega 3 are cofactors, and both are required for a healthy heart.

Congestive heart failure is caused by a single vitamin deficiency – thiamine – and we humans have known about this for at least 50 years, because this is what was killing dolphins and porpoises in captivity until Dr. Wallach figured out the problem. The animals were eating fish that contained an enzyme – thiaminase – that basically destroys thiamine. Since they were eating more of this enzyme than they were eating thiamine, they regularly died of congestive heart failure after only a short time in captivity. The solution was to change the types of fish being fed to captive mammals, and to supplement them with all the vitamins, including thiamine.

This problem is also understood in standard agriculture. A bull costs a farmer about $4,000-$5,000, and so it is a priority to keep the animal healthy for several breeding years. It makes no sense to let any animal die of congestive heart failure, because the cause and reversal is completely understood. The cost of correcting a thiamine deficiency in a bull, via a few thiamine injections, is less than $10. With a quick search online I found a 100ml container of injectable thiamine for $8.95. The recommended dose of that product is 0.25ml per 100 pounds of body weight for a large animal like a horse or cow. The first injection will probably save the animal's life, and for a 2,400 pound bull that $8.95 container provides over 16 injections appropriate to the body weight. That's a pretty good deal, and I think humans should take note of how cheap it can be to reverse a life-threatening problem like congestive heart failure.

The second reason foods can contribute to "heart disease", is because artery problems can be caused by food. You can see that it really doesn't make sense to lump all these problems together in one name, as congestive heart failure is very different from thrombotic stroke. Blood sugar problems and blood cholesterol problems tend to go hand in hand, and there is a definite, well-understood connection between blood sugar and a hardening of the cell membrane. The cell membrane is supposed to be "semi-permeable", meaning it lets some things into the cell, and some things out of the cell, selectively. The cell membrane is made partially of cholesterol, and when there is a blood sugar problem this cholesterol hardens, making it more difficult for things to get in and out of the cell. One of the consequences of this is more sugar and more cholesterol trapped in the blood, unable to be delivered into the cells.

We assume that it is not the blood sugar *causing* this membrane hardening, rather that both problems are caused by the same general nutrient deficiencies. In any case, when the body is unhealthy it can have either a blood sugar problem, or a blood cholesterol problem, or both. More cholesterol in the blood, in theory, will impact overall blood circulation. But this is not the real problem, as we see it. Several populations of people, such as the arctic Inuit (Eskimos), and the African Masai, eat much more cholesterol than the average westerner (the Inuit diet is almost *all* cholesterol), and yet these people do not die of what we call heart diseases. So high cholesterol itself is not a problem.

Carnivore animals do not get atherosclerosis (the buildup of fats on the artery walls), or arteriosclerosis (hardening of artery walls), but herbivore animals *do*. Especially herbivores in captivity. Our explanation for this is that these animals are largely eating *oxidized* grains and other foods. All foods will oxidize if they are left around in hot barrels and warehouses, and this tends to happen with big mammals who eat tons of food – the food sits around and it oxidizes. You can smell a batch of old peanuts or soy beans and tell immediately that something is off – the oils have turned rancid. Animals that eat this stuff will have an artery problem, and our explanation for this is free-radical damage to the insides of the veins. Foods are absorbed into the blood and free-radicals will impact the walls of the blood vessels. These animals do not eat cholesterol, and so it is silly to tell humans that their atherosclerosis or arteriosclerosis is caused by eating cholesterol when this is not what occurs in animals.

All of this is merely to say, in more detail than we covered in the book, that "the bad foods" cause much of what we call heart disease, and nutrient deficiencies cause the rest. This is why we recommend *both* avoiding the bad foods, *and* supplementing with all 90 essential nutrients. Humans who do so should avoid premature death from heart disease, stroke, and any of the vascular problems available.

Finally, I failed to mention dementias in the book. Alzheimer's disease was on the list of "good fat" diseases, but I didn't go into detail. Alzheimer's gets most of the attention these days, but it is definitely not the only form of dementia. The reason why Alzheimer's is on the good fat deficiency list is because the official problem in Alzheimer's is an unraveling of the "white matter" that coats all nerves. The white matter, the insulating material around the "wires" of nerves, is called "myelin." Alzheimer's is characterized by de-myelination, an unraveling of the myelin. Obviously, wires without insulation are a fire hazard, and it is a similar situation when our nerves lose their protective coating. Myelin is actually much more complicated than a mere insulation, as it is directly involved with the transmission of neurotransmitters and much more that is beyond the scope of this book. Problems with the nerves themselves or the myelin coating are also present in seizure disorders, and we give the same advice for any of the dementias that we would for any neurological problem.

Alzheimer's is in the spotlight these days, but technically Alzheimer's can only be properly diagnosed at autopsy, because we currently lack the ability to see the microscopic demyelination in a living patient. So, I assume that most Alzheimer's patients have actually been misdiagnosed, and the reason I say this is because the other dementias do not involve demyelination, and since demyelination takes a long time to develop, I assume most dementias are simpler nutrient deficiencies. The proof of this is if a patient is able to recover their memory and function in a short time – demyelination takes a long time to happen, and a long time to reverse (months, at least), and if a person recovers in a week, they definitely did not have Alzheimer's.

I assume that the most common form of dementia is actually "vitamin B12 deficiency dementia." I didn't make that name up, it's a real "disease." Just like the symptoms of "scurvy" appear with vitamin C deficiency, symptoms of dementia appear with deficiencies in several of the B vitamins, particularly B12. Humans have known about these vitamin deficiencies for hundreds of years, and I really don't know why it is barely ever mentioned that B vitamin deficiency can cause dementia. Doctors speak as if we have eradicated vitamin deficiency problems with our modern food fortification, but I see scurvy and rickets all the time in people at the grocery store. I also see dementia all the time, and the first thing I assume is a vitamin deficiency.

"Pellagra" is one of the oldest disease names that is still in use. Pellagra is the name for vitamin B3 (niacin) deficiency, and has always been described with "the three D's": diarrhea, dermatitis, dementia. The fourth D is *death*. I don't know why a doctor wouldn't want to cover this basic base before giving a diagnosis of Alzheimer's – if their patient got better quickly with a simple vitamin regimen, Alzheimer's could be safely ruled out.

This one vitamin deficiency is also known to cause several other problems that are mostly given separate disease names these days, without ever mentioning vitamin deficiency as a possible cause. Niacin deficiency can cause: sensitivity to sunlight, hair loss, swelling, tongue inflammation, trouble sleeping, weakness, mental confusion or aggression, ataxia (lack of coordination), paralysis of extremities, peripheral neuritis (nerve damage), enlarged or weakened heart, as well as various psychosensory and emotional disturbances. All of this is in regular textbooks about human and animal nutrition. A similar list could be drawn for every one of the vitamins, and the rest of the essential nutrients. The list above can be symptoms of many "diseases" with foreign-sounding Latin or German names, but chances are good that these symptoms and many others that are called "diseases" will simply go away with a decent supplement program, and avoiding foods like gluten that disrupt absorption of these nutrients. Many people report full recovery from these types of symptoms just by going gluten-free.

Alzheimer's and the other main dementias like Wernicke-Korsakoff dementia involve more serious structural damage than vitamin deficiency dementia. The human body is an absolute miracle of healing. The human body can live for decades on potato chips and soda, and it will use absolutely anything it can to get the job of repairing tissues done. In practice, people with dementia often rebound quite quickly when they are given the right advice and good supplements, and all of these I assume were simple vitamin and mineral deficiencies.

The vascular dementias like Wenicke-Korsakoff are more than simple deficiencies, because they are coupled with tissue damage. That tissue damage is from eating the bad foods we have discussed. The recommendation for these people is more than just avoiding the bad foods and taking the 90 essential nutrients – we also recommend consuming A LOT of cholesterol and other fatty foods that are not burned. This is because the nervous system, including the myelin, is made largely from cholesterol and the other good fats. The brain and nervous system are part of the "good fat" system, and so eating more good fat is a huge part of our advice. In addition, it is wise to boost the several key nutrients in this fat system, particularly selenium and the omegas.

Reversing dementia really can be that simple, but there is one more confounding factor that really gets in the way of this healing – statin drugs. Drugs that lower cholesterol actually stop the body from producing cholesterol and other essential functions. The body needs cholesterol – the body *makes* some of its own cholesterol.

Cholesterol has numerous vital roles, some of which have been mentioned, such as the cell membrane, and it is part of the structure of the nervous system. Cholesterol is also what the sex hormones and adrenal hormones are derived from. We can't synthesize vitamin D from sunlight without the cholesterol in our skin. There are many more essential roles of cholesterol, but the point here is that it is very important. When a person takes a drug that interferes with the cholesterol system, they will *inevitably* develop a "disease." One of those potential diseases is Alzheimer's. We call Alzheimer's a "physician-caused disease", because limiting cholesterol intake does almost nothing to blood cholesterol – doctors know this, and that is why they recommend cholesterol lowering drugs. Lowering cholesterol intake doesn't do much because the body will compensate for the deficiency by producing more cholesterol itself.

Along with other bad advice, such as avoiding salt, which is required to break fats down in the stomach before they go into the intestines for absorption, taking a cholesterol-lowering drug practically guarantees that some form of dementia will develop. Also practically guaranteed is another problem in the good fat system – skin, lungs, hormones, soft tissues all over the body, etc.

I have avoided going into detail about the harm that pharmaceutical drugs can potentially cause, because that topic deserves a book unto itself. Much of this book was about broad categories of disease, and we could have gone into great detail on any specific diseases, but they all fall into the categories we have discussed. By discussing these categories, a large part of the point was that pharmaceutical drugs are not appropriate for dealing with these types of problems. If drugs are unnecessary for dealing with chronic problems, then *any* harm caused by those drugs was also unnecessary.

Though this book was not about drugs, I do see the over-use of pharmaceuticals as one of the biggest problems in modern society. We already had it bad enough with a food system depleted of essential nutrients, and foods that physically harm us, but we have been put into a situation where we are nearly guaranteed to be even more harmed by seeking medical treatment for the problems caused by our foods and lack of nutrients.

All drugs have "side effects", including death. It is made to seem like these side effects are rare or unexpected, but based on the data of every drug, these really should just be called "effects", because they are normal consequences of consuming the drugs, and they are completely expected. Even drugs that can save our life, such as antibiotics, have expected, regular, negative effects on our bodies.

In my position, I know that the average person will have health problems, even with no history of pharmaceutical drug use. That is an expected outcome of eating modern foods and failing to consume all 90 essential nutrients. But I also know that anyone on any pharmaceutical drug should expect less progress with our nutritional strategies. If they are on the two worst types of drugs mentioned in the book – statin drugs and stomach acid lowering drugs – then I expect them to make no progress at all, no matter what they do, if they choose to stay on those drugs.

Legally we can't tell anyone to take or not take a drug, but we can talk about them, and I can give them my honest opinion that those two types of drugs will make it basically impossible for them to improve, even with the cleanest of eating and the best supplements in the world. We can talk about whether a drug has withdrawal concerns or not, but ultimately we have to encourage the person to work with their doctor(s) about lowering doses or stopping any drug. Most drugs, in our opinion, should be weaned, but the statins and stomach acid drugs have no benefit to weaning or withdrawal concerns. The stomach drugs will still stop the stomach from working properly, even in low doses, and so there is just no benefit to weaning – it will only prolong their misery. Statins, similarly, still work in low doses, and since there are no withdrawal concerns it simply doesn't make sense to do any other nutritional changes until the drug is stopped.

If a person is on multiple drugs of any type, I expect the person to continue to have health problems until they are weaned off. All the time we get people who tell us that many of their symptoms have improved with our advice, but they still have this or that thing bothering them. Most often, the person is still on some drug, even an over the counter NSAID or antihistamine. They want further advice from me about more things to do nutritionally, but I know that the problem is likely being caused by the drug, however innocuous it might seem.

Many people have speculated a connection between the rising prevalence of "female problems" like endometriosis and polycystic ovary syndrome to the use of chemical birth control in women, and I do agree. It is very common for women to come to us with "female problems", and tell us about a history of problems starting with their use of chemical birth control. I cannot quantify this properly, but in the very least, I do believe there is a connection. Logically it makes sense that messing with the hormone system could lead to problems in the hormone system, but unfortunately, young women are still prescribed birth control for all sorts of things having nothing to do with preventing a pregnancy. Women can be recommended birth control for reducing acne, regulating menstruation, and easing cramps. Acne is caused by eating the wrong foods or/and nutrient deficiencies, and irregular, light or heavy or painful menstruation are also caused by the same basic deficiencies.

All of these nutrient groups and symptom groups have been mentioned in this book – a lack or imbalance in the "good fats" is the most likely cause of any hormone or skin problem, and a deficiency in the bone/joint group is the most likely cause of any muscle or "pain" problem. Blood sugar problems can contribute to or cause any "female" problem, and I expect any woman with any of these problems to have an obvious blood sugar problem on their list of symptoms. None of this has anything to do with pharmaceuticals, and in my opinion it is at best criminally negligent for any professional to recommend chemical hormone disruption for a nutritional problem, leaving aside the actual issue of birth control.

Unfortunately, many people choose to listen to their doctors instead of apply basic nutritional changes and logic. I do sympathize with them, because we really are indoctrinated to believe that the doctor knows best. The reality is, of course, they often do not have a clue what causes, prevents, or reverses the problem in question. This is a tragedy on an unimaginable scale. We will always require medical professionals in emergency situations, but it is not emergencies that most of us go to a doctor for. We really can prevent and reverse most of the problems we can name, simply by being smart about our nutrition.

The best we can do for people who are involved with the medical system is to teach them the things in this book, and inform them that they are in fact in charge of what goes in and does not go into their body. They do not have to take anyone's advice. They do not have to take any drugs if they don't want to, and they can indeed get control of their health without any doctors.

One day medical doctors might be taught about nutrition, but I really wouldn't recommend waiting for this to happen on its own. For one thing, the payment structure would have to be changed. Doctors are paid, largely by insurance, for treating health problems. As outlined at the beginning of this book, treatment is done with drugs, tests, and surgeries. There simply isn't an existing framework for compensating medical doctors based on *preventing* diseases, or reversing them with nutritional strategies. We get paid on product sales, and doctors are not allowed to sell products. They're up against a wall, really. If they change their ways, they'll be broke. In any case, they aren't taught any of this, and I wouldn't expect the medical schools to completely change their way of thinking about diseases. It is up to *you* to change the way that you, your friends and your family understand and respond to diseases and health problems.

Similarly, I don't have hope in the "alternative" fields either. Naturopathic doctors are now essentially being trained the same as standard medical doctors. They are taught to largely rely on pharmaceuticals and surgeries, with some herbs and vitamins mixed in. They call this "mixed", or "complimentary" medicine, but really it is standard mainstream medicine with a tiny bit of nutrition or plant medicine involved. Though I believe that both allopathic and naturopathic systems are required for a balanced medical marketplace, I do not believe they "compliment" each other in most cases. If the antibiotic saves your life, you do need to replenish your good bacteria, which is in a sense "complimentary" – the two strategies are opposite but both necessary in this particular case.

Most other uses of pharmacology have no corresponding "complimentary" natural strategy – a statin drug will completely negate any benefit from doing the opposite, which is consuming cholesterol. If you take a statin, it eliminates any benefit from following my nutritional advice. There is no "mix" of benefits – you will get the harm from the drug, and no benefit from anything else. Similar statements could be made with practically any other drug type – a "beta blocker" stops the heart from working correctly, and it makes no sense to "support and promote a healthy heart" with nutrition while simultaneously using a drug that interferes with a healthy heart. I expect the person doing chemotherapy to die from the chemotherapy, regardless of any other "mixed" treatments, and so on through the list of available pharmaceutical treatments.

Even veterinarians are now prescribing drugs to dogs and cats to "manage" diabetes and arthritis, which are diseases they should have been taught are prevented with standard animal feeds. They should be giving pet owners the same advice we give our human customers – don't feel the animal human food, or it will get human diseases. All the essential nutrients for the animal are in the animal food designed for it, and human food throws off this balance. They should know this, but the modern animal and human practitioners of almost any name have been inculcated in the allopathic belief system. Allopathic medicine believes that humans, and now animals, are simply bags of bones waiting to break. They believe that the best way to "manage" this inevitable deterioration is with pharmaceutical drugs and surgeries.

This belief is unfortunate, but fortunately, you do not have to believe it yourself.

Acknowledgments.

All of the core information in this book derives from Dr. Joel Wallach's work. I credit him with my health, because his products got me out of pain, and his protocols have allowed me to optimize and thrive.

On top of the nutritional information, Dr. Wallach is a leader in this field of personal health, and he is the reason I am on this mission too. There are few people on Earth deserving the level of respect I have for him, and I will promote this message in his name as long as I am able to. My time with him not only taught me the protocols, but how to handle questions from the public.

Dr. Wallach has many books and lectures published and I recommend all of them.

I must also acknowledge Pharmacist Ben Fuchs as a core inspiration for the delivery of this message. He really helped me understand the human application of Dr. Wallach's message, and his generosity and support has been key to my growth in this field. I have stolen many key phrases and explanations from him.

Ben produces a lot of content and it can be found on www.PharmacistBen.com.

Another person I've borrowed heavily from is Dr. Peter Glidden. Dr. Glidden has done perhaps more than anyone in really breaking down the message. In the early days, we would meet someone with a health problem, then go home and watch a Dr. Glidden webinar on that problem.

Not only does Dr. Glidden go into great detail on what causes diseases, he explains what works and what doesn't and why. More importantly, he explains how and why to talk about these things legally. My main understanding about the legal importance of *disease, treatment* and *cure,* come from Dr. Glidden's teaching.

Dr. Glidden has a YouTube channel *Glidden Healthcare,* and you can find more about him on www.Glidden.Healthcare.

Dr. Glidden has two books: *The MD Emperor Wears No Clothes,* and *Attempt a Cure With Holistic Medicine.*

I am not sure if I can name our company next to the specific claims I've made in this book, but I will acknowledge what I think of as the family business. I have met so many amazing people in this business, and many of them have given me their time, advice, books, and other forms of support. I cannot name them all and I cannot properly express my gratitude to everyone who has helped me in this journey.

Outside of our company I have found warmth and support in the alternative health world as well. Many big names in the business carry a respect for Dr. Wallach, and my association with him has granted me access to some people you would normally have to wait in line to meet. Many great people promote many different pathways to health in this field, and I don't find that much competition. Most of us have our own turf, and even competing products generally share a respect for other companies. I have become friends with several people in other companies and have learned a lot from them. We all share common goals of promoting good health information.

I'm proud to work in this field and in this company. I don't know where I would be without this information, and I hope it has helped any reader reach a better understanding.

I would also like to acknowledge the many people who have supported me in my growth as an "influencer" online. It is you in the audience who keep me in check, hone my ability to explain things, and generally keep me going. I probably would have given up the very difficult task of teaching all of this stuff if it weren't for you guys. It is because of you that I know the difference our efforts make, and it is because of you that I will not stop.

I have mentioned that my mother is my biggest supporter, but she has done far more than encouragement. I haven't always been a good per-son or a good son, but she has always stuck by me. In my darkest years, she was always there to talk to, even when I didn't have anything good to say. Now she is practically my best friend, and I couldn't be more grateful. On top of all of that, she handles much of our shipping these days, which she is not compensated for nearly enough.

Finally, my lovely wife is easily my toughest critic, and without her keeping me sharp I may get lazy in my presentation. It is because of her that my books are thoroughly researched and edited, and it is for our life together that I work so tirelessly for.

From the bottom of my heart, thank you all.

146

About the Author.

I was born in Toronto, Ontario, Canada. I have no college or university degrees. I have lived in 5 countries on 4 continents, introduce myself as an artist or a marketer, and am an avid reader. I intend eventually to come up with some kind of title implying my work in healthcare, though for now my primary job is to creatively market health information.

I first learned about supplementation in my high school years, operating an exotic pet business, involving the breeding of the exotics and the feeder animals. I learned about nutrition and fitness as an employee and shift manager at Excel Fitness, in Pickering, Ontario, Canada.

I learned how to conduct proper scientific experiments, variable research, and data analysis while working in CO2 mitigation through ocean fertilization, with the Ocean Technology Group at the University of Sydney, Australia, and the Sydney Institute for Marine Science. My primary sponsor and mentor was Dr. Ian S. F. Jones, to whom I owe a great deal of my critical thinking. I have also worked on coral conservation in the Pacific waters of Costa Rica.

In 2015 my life-long health challenges were quickly reversed using Dr. Wallach's protocols. I have been promoting the message ever since.

I currently live half-time in Kirkland Lake, Ontario, and the other half in Spring, Texas, and work full time producing health-based content for the internet and answering the questions it produces. I plan to carry on Dr. Wallach's role of continuous speaking, and am open to invitations.

Recommended Reading.

The following recommendations are in alphabetical order and pertain to subjects referenced in the book.

- *The Biology of Belief: Unleashing the Power of Consciousness, Matter & Miracles* – B. H. Lipton.

Lipton is known as one of the "fathers of epigenetics", which is the science of how genes are affected by the environment and nutrition. This book goes into particular detail on the power of the human mind to influence the health of the body. Lipton not only goes into great detail about the science of epigenetics, but also details several incredible cases of disease reversal with the mind alone.

- *The Case Against Fluoride: How Hazardous Waste Ended Up in Our Drinking Water and the Bad Science and Powerful Politics That Keep it There* – P. Connett, J. Beck.

The issue of fluoride is more than just a question of health benefit or harm. Fluoride was the first and most widespread "medicine" that was given to entire populations of people against their will. This bypassed the long-established right of "informed consent", which makes it a particularly important case to understand. Whether fluoride is good or not, (and the book makes an excellent case that it is not good), fluoride is given to us for a medical purpose – preventing tooth decay. Since we are supposed to give our informed consent to ingest medications, this is a very important history to understand. Powerful politics have indeed acted against us in at least two ways: harming us with harmful medication, and bypassing our right to consent. This is definitely the best book on this subject that I know of.

• *Chasing the Cure: An Effective Alternative for Treating Cancer and Other Diseases* – W. Bengston, S. Fraser.

I haven't found that many books in the category of "faith healing" that I am able to recommend, but I really enjoyed this one and I think everyone should know about the possibility of spontaneous healing, without medication *or* nutrition. I believe we should use all healing modalities available, but faith and the inner placebo response are often left out of our mechanical approaches to health problems. I can recommend all the nutrition that I know, but I also know that your mind is more powerful than any treatment, and there are plenty of cases, some of which are described in this book, where the person healed with no other treatment other than someone who believed they could help you heal. Part of why I like this book more than other faith-based books is that the author participated in several experiments with mice, which is very interesting and I think speaks deeply to the power of the mind to heal.

• *The Cholesterol Myths: Exposing the Fallacy That Saturated Fat and Cholesterol Cause Heart Disease* – U. Ravnskov.

This book goes into incredible detail about the long history of misleading science behind the cholesterol scare. The medical establishment has no idea what causes, prevents, or reverses heart problems, and so they have looked for things to blame. Cholesterol and saturated fat have bore the brunt of their efforts to explain heart disease, but as this book clearly shows, the science involved is hardly convincing.

• *Deadly Medicines and Organised Crime: How Big Pharma Has Corrupted Healthcare* – P. C. Gøtzsche.

Gøtzsche goes into great detail on the harm of pharmaceuticals, and the length to which the pharmaceutical industry has manipulated data and public perception in order to sell their drugs. This is probably the most thorough book that I know of covering the demonstrated harm of pharmaceuticals.

- *Dissolving Illusions: Disease, Vaccines, and the Forgotten History* – S. Humphries, R. Bystrianyk.

This is by far the most detailed book that I know of on the history and harms of vaccines. Most people think that vaccines have eradicated many diseases, but this book comes as close to what I think is possible in proving that this is not true. The harm of vaccines has been buried since the very beginning of their use, and there is convincing evidence, thoroughly outlined in this book, that the disease disappearances credited to vaccines were in fact due to improved hygiene, and the renaming of diseases.

- *The Dorito Effect: The Surprising New Truth About Food and Flavor* – M. Schatzker.

This book isn't as scientifically-oriented as others on this list, but I highly enjoyed learning about the chemical manipulation of our foods that have the aim of getting us to eat more. It is already bad enough that the base ingredients of modern foods are mostly bad, but the situation is made much worse by the manipulation of flavors. The food industry is more insidious than I knew, and I recommend this book because it made me see processed foods in an even darker light.

- *Epigenetics: The Death of the Genetic Theory of Disease Transmission* – J. Wallach, M. Lan, G. N. Schrauzer.

This book goes through the entire history of failed theories about the origins of diseases, as well as outlining our modern understanding of the nutritional relationship to genes. Epigenetics is the science of how genes are affected by the environment, including nutrition, and I know of no better book for describing the concepts involved.

- *Grain Brain: The Surprising Truth About Wheat, Carbs, and Sugar – Your Brain's Silent Killers* – D. Perlmutter.

This is one of my favorite books outlining the scientifically-demonstrated harm that wheat and other grains do to the human body, and specifically the brain.

- *The Health Benefits of Tobacco: The Surprising Therapeutic Effects of Moderate Smoking and Second Hand Smoke* – W. C. Douglass II.

Since writing *Fake Diseases* I have tried to read every book I could find that disagrees with the anti-smoking crusade. Before this reading binge, I thought, like most people probably think, that the case against tobacco was as clear as a case could be. I had no idea how many outright lies and frauds were involved. I had no idea that science could be manipulated for political purposes – I thought only pharmaceutical companies would manipulate data. I wanted to include at least one book that is "pro" tobacco on this recommended reading list, because it is a subject that most people take for granted. We all assumed that smoking was simply bad, and that was the end of it. But there is quite a lot more to say on the subject, and Douglass is both a medical doctor, and a smoker, and so unlike most of the authors I have read on the subject, I feel he is doubly qualified to go through the science and present a case for an actual *benefit* to tobacco use.

We have no reason to credit the government or mainstream medical science with understanding smoking, as they do not even understand heartburn. They needed something to blame for cancer and heart disease and many other diseases, and they have misled all of us with statistics and fraudulent science and advertisements to believe that they have figured out why we have these diseases. Smoking has decreased dramatically in response to the multi-decade fear campaigns about smoking, and yet the diseases smoking is blamed for have hardly decreased, or have increased. Clearly, smoking is not the explanation, and Douglass is a great place to start in understanding that.

- *The Invisible Rainbow: A History of Electricity and Life* – A. Firstenberg.

This is currently my favorite book going into the details of the harm of electromagnetic frequencies. I have been in the anti-EMF business for several years, but even I didn't know how bad the problem was, and how far the evidence of this harm stretched back – to the very first experiments with electricity and batteries. Prior to reading this book, I thought the main species affected by EMF was humans, but Firstenberg shows ample evidence for the harm to plants and animals as well. The mainstream still treats EMF like only kooks and quacks believe it is a problem, but Firstenberg presents a veritable mountain of evidence from scientists all over the world and spanning over a hundred years. This is a must read for understanding the scale of the EMF problem.

- *Misconceptions About the Causes of Cancer* – L. S. Gold, T. H. Slone, N. B. Manle, B. N. Ames.

This short book is an excellent overview of the problems with the statistical probabilities of many supposed influences on cancer. You might have noticed that *Fake Diseases* hardly mentioned common chemicals and other things that the general public and news media believes contributes to cancer. The reason for omitting these chemicals is that their contributions are hardly well-established, and this book is great for understanding that.

- *Nutrition and Physical Degeneration* – W. A. Price.

This is one of my all-time favorite books. Price went all over the world looking for people who had not yet been in contact with modern foods. What he compiled was a data set that will probably never be replicated, because these groups are now fully affected by modern agriculture. Price documented the direct relationship between eating modern foods and physical degeneration. He was looking for the cause of cavities, but he found that the same nutritional factors that caused cavities also caused most of the health problems we deal with in the modern world. He documented people who had never eaten modern foods, and compared them with people of the same genetic and cultural stock who had begun eating modern flours and sugars. He also documented several reversals of cavities and other health problems with simple nutritional changes. Price did his work before the age of supplements, and I always recommend this book for anyone trying to understand the relationship between food and health.

- *Our Daily Meds: How the Pharmaceutical Companies Transformed Themselves Into Slick Marketing Machines and Hooked the Nation on Prescription Drugs* – M. Petersen.

This large book goes into great detail on the ubiquity of pharmaceutical companies in our everyday lives, particularly in America. While other books go into the specific detail on the harm of pharmaceuticals, this book is more about the lengths to which pharmaceutical companies have inserted themselves into every aspect of our lives, and the lives of our children. The actual harm of pharmaceuticals, to me, is bad enough, but this book details how much deeper and darker these companies can be.

- *Passive Smoke: The EPA's Betrayal of Science and Policy* – G. B. Gori, J. C. Luik.

This short book examines the highly influential 1993 EPA report which condemned second-hand tobacco smoke as a cause of cancer and other diseases. The average person would think that the science behind tobacco smoke was clear and demonstrates an obvious risk to health. If that were the case, the EPA wouldn't have had to commit scientific fraud to make their case. A lot of policy has been built on the anti-smoking campaign, and so it is very important that we understand just how much manipulation was involved in creating the public image that smoking was the cause of a long list of diseases. Like cholesterol, the medical world has no idea what causes, prevents, or reverses cancer or heart disease or the many other health problems that smoking takes the blame for. They had to blame something, and they have used weak statistical correlations and other forms of data manipulation to make their case. Smoking policy has been created "for our own good", and this same framework has been used to implement the many new laws and mandates we have experienced since 2020. Bogus data can lead to real government policies that affect us all.

- *The Peanut Allergy Epidemic: What's Causing it and How to Stop it* – H. Fraser.

I didn't cover allergies in *Fake Diseases* because it can be quite complicated. Many people refer to environmental sensitivities like "hay fever" with the word "allergy", but a sensitivity to pollen or cat hair or the occurrence of "seasonal allergies", are not actual allergies. Real allergies cause a serious reaction, are life-threatening, and require an injection of epinephrine. Real allergies are a bit of a mystery to both mainstream and alternative medicine, but this book makes a detailed and interesting case that many of our current allergies are caused by ingredients in vaccines. I highly recommend this book, even though I do not think it explains *all* allergies, it does, to me, explain many of them.

- *The Placebo Response: How You Can Release Your Body's Inner Pharmacy For Better Health* – H. Brody.

Positive results with nutritional or spiritual strategies are often denounced as "the placebo effect." The mind is indeed one of the most powerful, if not *the* most powerful tool for healing available. We all should understand this phenomenon, rather than using it as a way to dismiss results. This book doesn't have all the answers, but gives a lot of information about how we can all maximize our body's natural ability to heal itself. For those of us promoting health products and protocols, it is very useful for us to be able to call upon all the most effective tools for bringing out the placebo response in addition to the active methods we are employing with a client. I highly recommend this book to anyone attempting to heal themselves or others. We cannot dismiss the placebo effect, we have to work with it.

- *Rare Earths, Forbidden Cures* – J. Wallach, M. Lan.

This book is the most detailed overview of the relationship between nutrients and diseases that I know of. This type of detail is normally found in textbooks, but *Rare Earths* is publicly available and written for a general audience. It includes a lot of documented evidence as well as examples from standard media to draw the connections between nutritional deficiencies and diseases and causes of death.

- *Sit Less: Evolve Your Work and Life Without Compromising Your Health* – S. Zavalin.

This has recently become one of my favorite books on the subject of movement. Rather than emphasizing full-on exercise, Zavalin takes a very realistic approach to helping those of us who sit for a living to improve our health with simple steps revolving around sitting less. I know that the average person does not have to go to a gym to get healthy, and that exercise itself is not *the* key factor to health, but we are definitely designed to move, and we modern people definitely tend to sit way too much. This book is short and very practical, and I recommend it for all chronic sitters.

- *Wheat Belly: Lose the Wheat, Lose the Weight, and Find Your Path Back to Health* – W. Davis.

One of the questions that comes up when I say that gluten is bad is: "why is it any different now than it was in the Bible, or for my grandmother." Wheat has changed significantly since ancient times, and even since the time of our grandparents. This is my favorite book for outlining the history of wheat, and similar grains, and the demonstrated harm that modern grains have done to us.

- *Zapped: Why Your Cell Phone Shouldn't Be Your Alarm Clock and 1,269 Ways to Outsmart the Hazards of Electrical Pollution* – A. L. Gittleman.

This is my current favorite book outlining many practical strategies that we can implement to reduce the effect of EMF in our daily lives. Other books go into great detail on the actual science of the harm, but fail to give us many practical suggestions for reducing the harm. This book is very accessible and requires no technical knowledge of EMF.

More.

@WallachsWarriors is our main Instagram account. We regularly answer live audience questions and we will answer every message in the inbox.

Our products can be found at www.WallachsWarriors.ca. We encourage you to contact us for help figuring out what might be best for you. As well as any of the accounts listed, you can email us at YGYOntario@gmail.com.

We also have an Instagram page for more detailed nutritional information @WarriorsAdvanced, and a page for personal development and sales training material @WallachsDistributors.

@NotusFoods teaches how to make practically every dish you could think of without the bad foods listed. We have talented cooks and bakers who will take requests and answer questions. We also have a YouTube channel *Notus Foods* to teach cooking according to our guidelines.

@RyanAleckszander is my personal Instagram account and I post mostly book reviews. My personal YouTube channel is *TheRealNotus,* where I post mostly my opinion, as well as read-along versions of my books.

I also have a podcast, *Notus & Friends.*

@TranscendTowers is my cellphone tower Instagram account, as well as miscellaneous conspiracy material.

@TheRealNotus is my art Instagram account. Behind everything else, I was always supposed to be an artist. I also have a YouTube channel

Notus Art, teaching art on a budget.
I have art for sale at www.NotusArt.com

All of my books, audiobooks, and links are available at
www.NotusBooks.org.

We can be reached by phone, toll free in the USA. 1-888-211-2549.

Our cookbook teaches everything you would need to know to cook
without the bad foods.

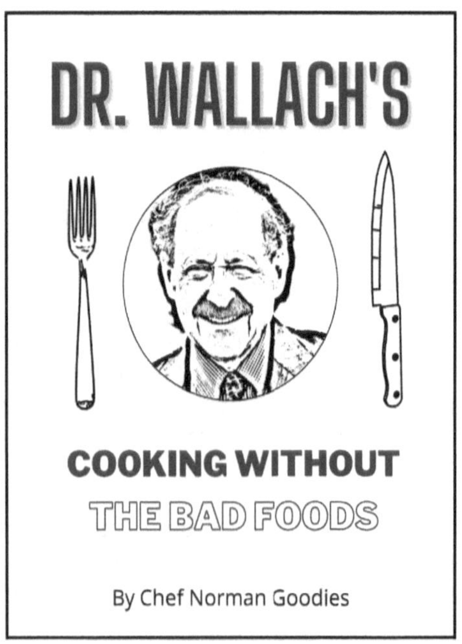

Dr Wallach's Cooking Without The Bad Foods
by Chef Norman Goodies | Jun 14, 2021
★★★★★ ⌄ 4
Paperback
$29⁹⁹

I have published a book in defense of Dr. Wallach, in response to his critics.

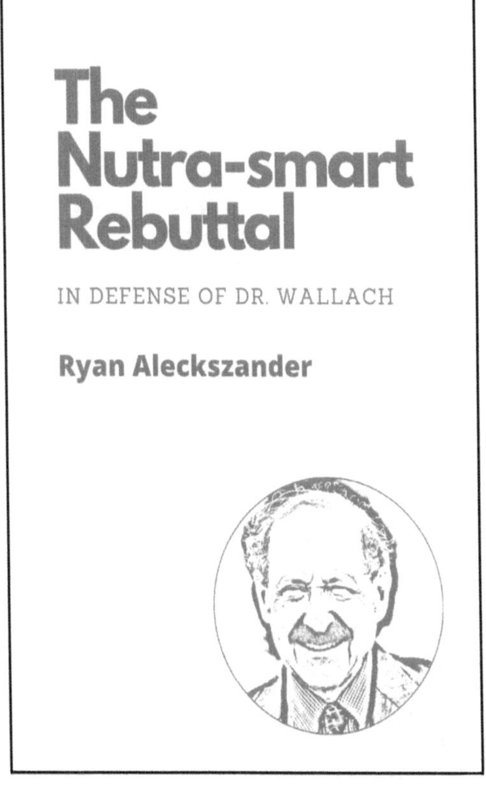

Nutri-smart rebuttal: in
defence of Dr. Wallach
by Ryan Aleckszander

Paperback
$9.99

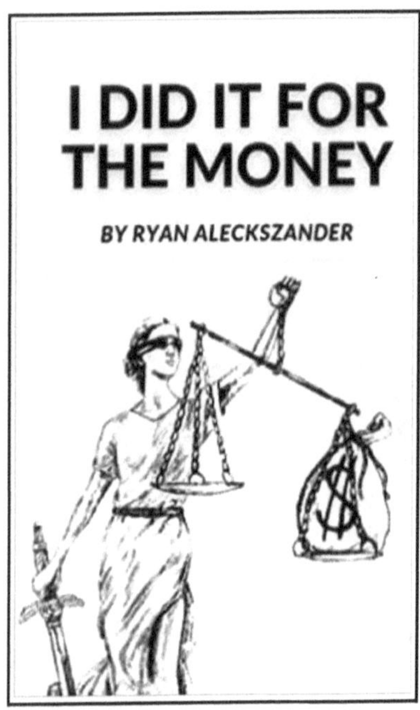

I Did It For The Money

by Ryan Aleckszander　|　Jun 10, 2021

Paperback

$7⁹⁹

I have attempted to run several businesses that were more about my heart than my head. These businesses failed.

Money must be one of the central goals in our lives, if we expect to adequately care for ourselves and our families. If we want to make a wider difference in the world, this is even more true.

I spent much of my life in poverty, and in this book I go through my financial life story leading to my eventual success.

I have used financial principles that have existed for centuries, and you can too.

There is an extended version of this book that includes my favorite financial story *The Richest Man In Babylon*, by George Clason. It is only available in Canada and Japan. It costs a few dollars more and you can find those links on www.NotusBooks.org.

I have two separate problems with the government. Most of what governments do can be handled less expensively by private companies, and governments often do things that do not need to be done. Both cases are harmful, though to much different degrees.

In this book I discuss government failures in several categories including; infrastructure, food, health, environment, business, education, and more. Though I do not claim to have answers to all of the problems in these categories, I have some ideas for improvements.

Media and private conversations tend to attribute government failures to accidents, ignorance, arrogance, or that it was an isolated incident. Instead, I argue that these failures are predictable outcomes to government structure and policies.

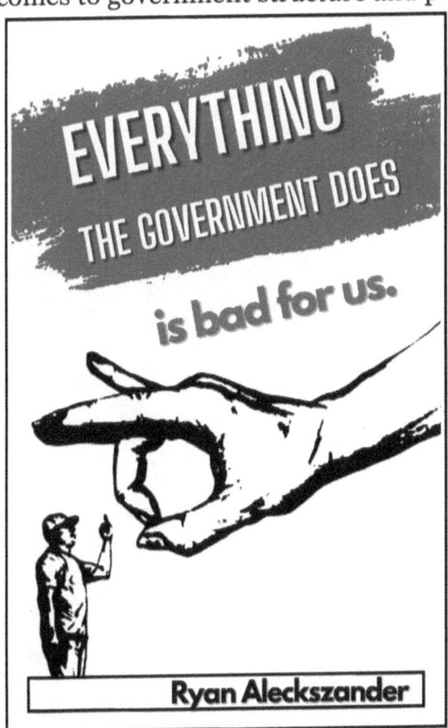

I believe there is a better way, but to have that conversation, first we must understand that everything the government does is bad for us.

Everything the Government Does is Bad For Us
by Ryan Aleckszander | Aug 18, 2021

Paperback Hardcover
$9⁹⁹ $15⁹⁹

Alphabetical Index

i   My understanding of pathology and pathogenesis of disease comes mostly from Dr. Joel Wallach. I don't mean this book to be academic, so I am not going to give citations for every disease. I encourage referencing Dr. Wallach's work for specific technical explanations about diseases.

ii   Thalassemia and sickle cell are the same thing under the microscope. Sickle cell is the name they give it when it appears in black people, thalassemia in white people. I assume this is because they believe this disease is genetically transmitted. We believe it is a birth defect, completely preventable like all other birth defects. And people with these problems can live a relatively healthy, long life, by following healthy lifestyle practices.

iii   USA Federal Register/ Vol. 78, No. 73 / Tuesday, April 16, 2013

iv   Vitamin and omega deficiencies are also common. And can cause misery. Plants can make vitamins, amino acids, essential fatty acids (omegas), antioxidants, and all kinds of medicinal compounds. But they can't make minerals. If minerals are not in the soil, they're not in the plant.

v   I like to use colloidal silver on wounds or fresh tattoos, after washing with unscented antibacterial soap.

vi   Actually there is a growing trend for pet owners to have insurance for their animals. Unfortunately, the veterinary world is being trained basically like human doctors now. They no longer understand how to prevent and reverse the common problems of diabetes and arthritis and so on in animals. Farmers still know this, for they *must* understand prevention or they will not be profitable – a wealthy dog owner might be able to afford pet insurance, but a farmer definitely could not operate that way.

vii   *Let's Play Doctor* (1989) is still the best source for specific disease explanations according to Dr. Wallach.

viii   Muscular dystrophy was first mentioned as white muscle disease in animals. We know this is caused by a selenium deficiency in pregnancy. But there are many cofactors involved. Selenium is a fat soluble mineral, and so it appears on the fat-deficiency problem list as well, because a cofactor deficiency will likely lead to several possible selenium deficiency problems.

ix   The best advice I can give is to do the salt flush as much as needed, and use digestive enzymes for a while (1-3 months). You might feel like doing the salt flush every day (see page 37). If there is stomach pain, salty water should help. But the longer you have been on the PPI's, the more sensitive your stomach will likely be.

Your digestive enzyme product should contain more than enzymes – it should also contain bile and a chloride compound like betaine HCl. We do sell more than one good enzyme product at www.WallachsWarriors.ca, in the digestion support category.

You also might want to fast a lot and do a lot of your meals in liquid. Bone broth made at home, vegetable broth, vegetable juices, fruit juices, liquid supplements, aloe, and fermented foods will be your best friends during this process.

There is not much more that you can do other than load your body up with liquid nutrients and let time pass.

x   There is an exception here that I should mention. The body may be prevented from actually getting the stomach acid into the stomach if there is osteoporosis pinching the vagus nerve in the back. So, some rare stomach problems are actually a back problem. The raw material needed to rebuild the spinal cord is the bone & joint group, covered in the bone & joint chapter.

xi Quinoa might seem out of place on my "definitely not" list, but it is there for good reason. When we tell people to pretend they are celiac, they will see quinoa on internet lists of permissible grains. I know from experience that this can still be a problem. Many people tell me they are "completely gluten-free", but on further investigation, they have replaced many of their grain-based dishes with quinoa, and are still showing signs of gluten intolerance. In other words, as long as they are eating quinoa they cannot seem to heal.

The most obvious of these signs is a lack of progress in their overall health, weight, skin, and so on. If they're not improving, there is still a problem, and since this happened so many times, I have banned quinoa for my clients. I do not see this with rice or teff or the others that are not on my "definitely avoid" list.

After you have completely "reset" your digestion, and have improved significantly over a period of *at least* three months, you can have a small bit of quinoa now and then, if you absolutely must. You can see if you have a direct reaction to it with a simple "pulse test." Do not eat for 24 hours, then eat only the suspect food. Take your pulse a few minutes before eating it, during, a few minutes after, and about an hour after. Write down the numbers, and if the pulse spiked significantly after eating the food, your body does not like it.

You can try the pulse test again in a couple of months, after even more internal healing has taken place, and there is a chance that the food is no longer a problem for you. You can do this for any food you suspect is aggravating your system – this is essentially a simpler version of the "elimination diet."

The above paragraph only counts for whole-grain quinoa. I do not ever recommend eating "gluten-free" products that use quinoa flour. When grains were milled with a stone, they were invariably much bigger pieces than the very finely-ground powders we get today by heavy equipment milling. Smaller particles have more surface area. Our intestines are lined with villi and micro villi to expand surface area for absorption, which is a good thing. When bigger grain particles passed through the intestine, there was less chance that they would be absorbed into the blood, and there was less surface area on each particle, so there was less area to contact the villi and cause the contact enteritis (inflammation of the villi). Modern flours are much more finely ground, and therefore have much more surface area to irritate the guts.

xii   This can actually get more complicated, as mentioned in endnote x. A strong stomach acid is required to absorb most of the minerals, including calcium. Calcium is involved in all muscle contractions. It is muscle contractions of the chief cells in the stomach, which squirt the acid into the stomach.

So salt deficiency can contribute to the mineral deficiency of the mineral responsible for squirting the acid into the stomach. This is to get me off the hook if salt alone doesn't eliminate someone's stomach pain. There are more components to stomach acid, and more nutrients involved in getting the acid where it needs to be. This is why we recommend all of the essential nutrients, including NaCl, and Ca.

xiii   I didn't find space to mention colon hydrotherapy in the main text. Many people promote various kinds of enemas. We do not promote them for health reasons. Enemas clean the rectal cavity. This is fine to do, but the plaque buildup is going to be mostly in the colon.

I recommend colon hydrotherapy because I saw it remove plaque from me that years of good digestion and nutrition were not able to get rid of. I had practised everything else mentioned but I still had plaque in my colon.

Colon hydrotherapy should be done by a professional and it is not the cheapest therapy in the book. But it is comparable to the price of massage or chiropractic care. Regular interval sessions are recommended for best results. If you choose to do it, be prepared to do multiple sessions over a few months.

The hydrotherapist you choose should also be a kind and gentle person. You should have a good feeling about them. This person will be in a small room with you with a hose up your butt for up to an hour.

I have only used one practitioner, but I recommend her. Colorado Colonics & Detox Center. Currently in Englewood CO. They also offer sound/frequency therapy and I think it's great.

xiv   There are too many to properly cite. Every "qualified health claim" granted by the FDA has a large and solid body of evidence involved in the case.

xv   Chemists might not appreciate my simplicity in this description. Several of the compounds responsible for foods on our bad list have their own names like acrylamide or hetercyclic amines, or trans fatty acids. I am calling it all "free-radical damage" for simplicity.

xvi In the time since this book was first published I have been on a bit of a binge reading all the books I can find that disagree with the mainstream opinion that smoking causes basically all diseases. I didn't know about the problems in the research or the politically motivated campaign against smoking, but it turns out there is a lot more to the story than we are led to believe. I have included a couple of books on this subject in the recommended reading section, and I intend to write a book on it myself in the near future.

xvii   Bad list:

- Gluten (wheat, barley, rye), oats, quinoa.

Rice is probably okay but grain-free is probably best. We don't want a grain-based lifestyle.

- Liquid oils, heated oils, old oxidized fatty foods such as nuts or peanuts, deep-fried foods, burned butters, burned animal fats, well done red meat.

- Meats processed with nitrates/nitrites or a celery product.

- Carbonated drinks.

- Baked potato skins.

- Non organic soy or corn.

Every person could have foods that are not on this list which do not agree with their body. An "elimination diet" will help you find any of these.

The "diet" we recommend is close to "keto." The general recommendation is to eat more protein and fat than carbohydrates and sugar. Fruits and vegetables are all fine and good and there are only some technicalities that will matter if you are trying to optimize.

Our food instagram @NotusFoods is hosted by talented cooks and bakers and will answer any questions in the inbox.

xviii   *Zapped: why your cell phone shouldn't be your alarm clock and 1,268 ways to outsmart the hazards of electronic pollution*, is my favorite pratical handbook on how to reduce this stress in your life. By Ann Gittleman.

xix   We are not allowed to diagnose people with a disease, but we can ask them about their existing health problems. Some of these questions can change our recommendations, such as a missing gallbladder, or the presence of a stomach acid lowering drug, or shellfish allergy.

I have made content describing the process of asking and answering these questions on our YouTube channel *Wallach's Warriors,* and my podcast *Notus & Friends.*

Here is the questionnaire we are currently using:

- Age/height/weight/sex/country:

- All symptoms, all diagnoses:

- Have they had any surgeries? Any organs or glands removed?

- Are they on any chemical drugs?

- Do they take any supplements? Herbs or natural medicines?

- Do they avoid any foods? Do they have any sensitivities? Allergies?

- Do they have any skin, lung, or digestive issues?

- Do they know their blood type?

- Any sleeping problems? Teeth grinding or sweating at night? Nightmares?

- Were they born C sectioned?

- Are they pregnant or nursing or trying?

- Do they drink anything carbonated?

- Do they drink coffee or energy drinks?

- **Optional** – show us a picture of their finger or toe nails, not polished.

- What is their favorite food?

- Anything else we should know about?

Most of these questions can be expected on a form from a dentist office the first time you want to use their services. They do need some basic information to handle you properly. We can't prescribe drugs but we should know if you're on any.

xx   I sell a few anti EMF devices, including that patch, and frequency-tuning discs. www.WallachsWarriors.ca

xxi   Pesticides and herbicides and fungicides can nullify much of this process. As a result, plants grown in "non-organic" agriculture will have less minerals, and less overall nutritional value per carbohydrate.

The BRIX score is commonly used to measure the nutritional value of fruits and vegetables and berries. BRIX scores are invariably lower with non-organic crops, and invariably higher with additional colloidal minerals added. This can be experimented in any garden.

We sell the raw form of our human mineral supplement as garden fertilizer.

You might find this interesting: in the agriculture world, you can't pitch a farmer that he will increase his yields by more than 50%. You will sound like a lunatic to the farmer, and he will not take you seriously. They already have very impressive yields in modern agriculture with standard fertilizers focusing on Nitrogen, Phosphorus, and Potassium (NPK).

So, we are taught not to attempt to sell our plant derived mineral fertilizers with the numbers we are actually able to produce. We can achieve much more than 50% yield improvement on probably every crop imaginable.

xxii   My favorite books about gluten and grains are *Wheat Belly* by Dr. William Davis, and *Grain Brain* by Dr. David Perlmutter.

I would also include further reading on flour and sugar to include *Nutrition and Physical Degeneration* by Dr. Weston A. Price. This book is one of the classics and one of the bibles when it comes to natural healing and lifestyles.

xxiii   I would honestly add money deficiency to the "most common" stress list. It is no wonder that poorer people have more diseases generally. It is very stressful to be lacking in money or the life necessities that money buys.

xxiv   *Dissolving Illusions* by Suzanne Humphries is my favorite book on the subject. *Anyone Who Tells You Vaccines Are Safe And Effective Is Lying*, by Vernon Coleman, is my favorite recent read on the subject.

xxv The first denial was for attempting to volunteer at a farmer's market in America. I learned on that day that I am not allowed to contribute to the American economy in any way, without a work visa.

The second denial was for trying to bring a snake over the border without the requisite veterinary forms. I could have waited several hours for the border vet to arrive, but we chose to turn around, drop off the snake, and cross again that same night.

These incidents have not prevented me from being allowed to cross, but I do expect extra scrutiny.